Copyright © 2o20 by Brayden Shelley -All rights reserved.

No part of this publication may be reproduced, distributed, or transmitted in any form or by any means, including photocopying, recording, or other electronic or mechanical methods, without the prior written permission of the publisher, except in the case of brief quotations embodied in reviews and certain other non-commercial uses permitted by copyright law.

This Book is provided with the sole purpose of providing relevant information on a specific topic for which every reasonable effort has been made to ensure that it is both accurate and reasonable. Nevertheless, by purchasing this Book you consent to the fact that the author, as well as the publisher, are in no way experts on the topics contained herein, regardless of any claims as such that may be made within. It is recommended that you always consult a professional prior to undertaking any of the advice or techniques discussed within.This is a legally binding declaration that is considered both valid and fair by both the Committee of Publishers Association and the American Bar Association and should be considered as legally binding within the United States.

CONTENTS

INTRODUCTION 5
BREAKFAST AND BRUNCH RECIPES 6
    Ham & Hash Brown Casserole 6
    Tomato Quiche 7
    Eggs In Avocado Cups 8
    Bacon & Spinach Muffins 9
    Sausage With Eggs & Avocado 10
    French Toast Sticks 11
    Bell Pepper Omelet 12
    Baked Eggs 13
    Egg & Spinach Tart 14
    Tex-mex Hash Browns 15
    Breakfast Frittata 16
    Cheese Toasts With Eggs & Bacon 17
    Banana Bread 18
    Cinnamon And Sugar Doughnuts 19
    Roasted Cauliflower 20
    Sweet Potato Tots 21
    Garlic Cheese Bread 22
    Potato Rosti 23
FISH & SEAFOOD RECIPES 24
    Air Fryer Salmon 24
    Herbed Scallops 25
    Halibut & Shrimp With Pasta 26
    Spiced Tilapia 27
    Green Beans With Southern Catfish 28
    Herbed Salmon 29
    Grilled Fish Fillet In Pesto Sauce 30
    Prawn Burgers 31
    Zesty Fish Fillets 32
    Crusted Sole 33
    Crusted Salmon 34
    Pesto Salmon 35
    Seasoned Catfish 36
    Crumbed Fish 37
    Lemon Dill Mahi Mahi 38
    Glazed Salmon 39
    Cod Parcel 40
    Ranch Tilapia 41
POULTRY RECIPES 42
    Spicy Chicken Legs 42
    Herbed Turkey Breast 43
    Popcorn Chicken 44
    Bang-bang Chicken 45
    Asian Deviled Eggs 46

Roasted Cornish Game Hen...... 47
Seasoned Chicken Tenders...... 48
Herbed & Spiced Turkey Breast...... 49
Hard-boiled Eggs...... 50
Blackened Chicken Breast...... 51
Spiced Chicken Thighs...... 52
Lemony Turkey Legs...... 53
Air Fryer Chicken Wings...... 54
Thyme Duck Breast...... 55
Turkish Chicken Kebab...... 56
Herbed Roasted Chicken...... 57
Marinated Chicken Thighs...... 58
Glazed Turkey Breast...... 59

MEAT RECIPES...... 60
Bbq Baby Ribs...... 60
Buttered Leg Of Lamb...... 61
Mushrooms With Steak...... 62
Braised Lamb Shanks...... 63
Glazed Lamb Meatballs...... 64
Sweet Potato, Brown Rice, And Lamb...... 65
Buttered Rib Eye Steak...... 66
Beef Kabobs...... 67
Bacon-wrapped Filet Mignon...... 68
Stuffed Pork Roll...... 69
Almonds Crusted Rack Of Lamb...... 70
Ranch Pork Chops...... 71
Beef Chuck Roast...... 72
Lamb Sirloin Steak...... 73
Spiced Flank Steak...... 74
Italian-style Meatballs...... 75
Glazed Lamb Chops...... 76
Air-fried Meatloaf...... 77

VEGETARIAN AND VEGAN RECIPES...... 78
Broccoli With Cauliflower...... 78
Air Fryer Pumpkin Keto Pancakes...... 79
Basil Tomatoes...... 80
Buttered Veggies...... 81
Potato Tots...... 82
Corn Nuts...... 83
Green Beans & Mushroom Casserole...... 84
Veggie Kabobs...... 85
Sweet & Tangy Mushrooms...... 86
Spicy Potato...... 87
Glazed Mushrooms...... 88
Roasted Cauliflower And Broccoli...... 89
Potato-skin Wedges...... 90

- Baked Potatoes 91
- Spicy Butternut Squash 92
- Garlicky Brussels Sprout 93
- Spicy Green Beans 94
- Stuffed Pumpkin 95

SNACK & DESSERT RECIPES 96
- Air-fried Butter Cake 96
- Apple Fritters 97
- Crispy Coconut Prawns 98
- Cheddar Biscuits 99
- Vanilla Cheesecake 100
- Fried Pickles 101
- Chocolate Mug Cake 102
- Banana Split 103
- Gluten-free Cherry Crumble 104
- Glazed Figs 105

INTRODUCTION

Ninja Foodi

How does it work? Ninja Foodi has been tested to see if it can be used to prepare French fries, crunchy chicken, cheesecake, chicken patties, and other basic products in stand-alone pressure cookers and fryers.

Accessories Everywhere

The Foodi is selling for the 6.5-liter version between 1
90 and 230 US dollars, but the exact price depends on where you buy it. It sounds like lots of money, but you get a lot for that price.

One of the first things we noticed when Foodi arrived was that the capacity of the box is exceptionally high compared to instant pressure cookers and pressure cookers with similar cooking appliances. The fast cooking capacity of the Foodi is 6.5 liters, while the fryer can hold 4 liters.

When you open the big box, you'll find the Ninja Foodi oval hob with an air cooker lid and pressure cooker, as well as a sealing ring, a PTFE and PFOA-free ceramic tub, a cooking basket with air, an adjustable roasting pan. Side handles, condensate cup, cookbook, cooking instructions, and user guide.

Advantages Of Frying Without Oil (Air Fryer)

The traditional frying process involves introducing the food in a container with oil at high temperatures, between 150 and 200 ºC. The oil transmits the heat and quickly heats the ingredient and evenly.

This time we will talk about a new way of frying oil without food. Is it possible? Of course, you will see the explanation on how to do it and the advantages of this method:

How to fry without oil?

New air fryers on the market do not require oil or maybe just a little to cook food. They work with a system that incorporates hot air and takes advantage of the natural fat that fresh or frozen Ingredients have.

To obtain more crispy results, just add a spoonful of oil. Almost nothing compared to the amount used in a cheap conventional fryer.

With this technique, in addition to low caloric content, you will have rich dishes. You enjoy this crunchy texture but without the need to resort to large amounts of oil and, therefore, fats.

Advantages You Get When Frying Without Oil (Air Fryer)

Frying without oil is a way to enjoy crispy foods without falling into the use of too much oil. The advantages of the Air fryer are the following:

- Ideal to eat healthily. Calories decrease when using an air fryer because the amount of oil used is minimal or even nil.
- Food with rich flavor, in this form of cooking, do not give off odors. There is also no risk of the flavors mixing if you have already prepared another food with a strong flavor.
- Frying without oil does not allow food to oxidize, and there is no possibility that the oil will burn and become harmful.
- Cook and fry foods without messing everything up, free of oil splashes. When finished, it is much easier to clean the surroundings and the hot air fryer.

BREAKFAST AND BRUNCH RECIPES

Ham & Hash Brown Casserole

Servings: 5
Cooking Time: 35 Minutes

Ingredients:
- 1½ tablespoons olive oil
- ½ of large onion, chopped
- 24 ounces frozen hash browns
- 3 eggs
- 2 tablespoons milk
- Salt and freshly ground black pepper, to taste
- ½ pound ham, chopped
- ¼ cup Cheddar cheese, shredded

Directions:
1. In a skillet, heat the oil over medium heat and sauté the onion for about 4-5 minutes.
2. Remove from the heat and transfer the onion into a bowl.
3. Add the hash browns and mix well.
4. Place the mixture into a baking pan.
5. Press "Power Button" of Ninja Foodi Digital Air Fry Oven and turn the dial to select "Air Bake" mode.
6. Press "Time Button" and again turn the dial to set the cooking time to 32 minutes.
7. Now push "Temp Button" and rotate the dial to set the temperature at 350 degrees F.
8. Press "Start/Pause" button to start.
9. When the unit beeps to show that it is preheated, open the lid.
10. Arrange pan over the wire rack and insert in the oven.
11. Stir the mixture once after 8 minutes.
12. Meanwhile, in a bowl, add the eggs, milk, salt and black pepper and beat well.
13. After 15 minutes of cooking, place the egg mixture over hash brown mixture evenly and top with the ham.
14. After 30 minutes of cooking, sprinkle the casserole with the cheese.
15. When cooking time is complete, open the lid and place the casserole dish aside for about 5 minutes.
16. Cut into equal-sized wedges and serve.
17. Serving Suggestions: Avocado slices will accompany this casserole greatly.
18. Variation Tip: Use freshly shredded cheese.

Nutrition Info: Calories: 540 Fat: 29.8g Sat Fat: 6.5g Carbohydrates: 51.5g Fiber: 5.3g Sugar: 3.2g Protein: 16.7g

Tomato Quiche

Servings: 2
Cooking Time: 30 Minutes

Ingredients:
- 4 eggs
- ¼ cup onion, chopped
- ½ cup tomatoes, chopped
- ½ cup milk
- 1 cup Gouda cheese, shredded
- Salt, to taste

Directions:
1. In a small baking pan, add all the ingredients and mix well.
2. Press "Power Button" of Ninja Foodi Digital Air Fry Oven and turn the dial to select "Air Fry" mode.
3. Press "Time Button" and again turn the dial to set the cooking time to 30 minutes.
4. Now push "Temp Button" and rotate the dial to set the temperature at 340 degrees F.
5. Press "Start/Pause" button to start.
6. When the unit beeps to show that it is preheated, open the lid.
7. Arrange the pan over the wire rack and insert in the oven.
8. When cooking time is complete, open the lid and place the pan aside for about 5 minutes.
9. Cut into equal-sized wedges and serve.
10. Serving Suggestions: Fresh baby spring mix will be a great companion for this quiche.
11. Variation Tip: You can use any kind of fresh veggies for the filling of quiche.

Nutrition Info: Calories: 247 Fat: 16.1g Sat Fat: 7.5g Carbohydrates: 7.3g Fiber: 0.9g Sugar: 5.2g Protein: 18.6g

Eggs In Avocado Cups

Servings: 2
Cooking Time: 10 Minutes

Ingredients:
- 1 avocado, halved and pitted
- 2 large eggs
- Salt and freshly ground black pepper, to taste
- 2 cooked bacon slices, crumbled

Directions:
1. Carefully scoop out about 2 teaspoons of flesh from each avocado half.
2. Crack 1 egg in each avocado half and sprinkle with salt and black pepper lightly.
3. Arrange avocado halves onto the greased piece of foil-lined sheet pan.
4. Press "Power Button" of Ninja Foodi Digital Air Fry Oven and turn the dial to select "Air Roast" mode.
5. Press "Time Button" and again turn the dial to set the cooking time to 10 minutes.
6. Now push "Temp Button" and rotate the dial to set the temperature at 375 degrees F.
7. Press "Start/Pause" button to start.
8. When the unit beeps to show that it is preheated, open the lid and insert the sheet pan in the oven.
9. When cooking time is complete, open the lid and transfer the avocado halves onto serving plates.
10. Top each avocado half with bacon pieces and serve.
11. Serving Suggestions: Serve these avocado halves with cherry tomatoes and fresh spinach.
12. Variation Tip: Smoked salmon can be replaced with bacon too.

Nutrition Info: Calories: 300 Fat: 26.6g Sat Fat: 6.4g Carbohydrates: 9g Fiber: 6.7g Sugar: 0.9g Protein: 9.7g

Bacon & Spinach Muffins

Servings: 6
Cooking Time: 17 Minutes

Ingredients:
- 6 eggs
- ½ cup milk
- Salt and freshly ground black pepper, to taste
- 1 cup fresh spinach, chopped
- 4 cooked bacon slices, crumbled

Directions:
1. In a bowl, add the eggs, milk, salt and black pepper and beat until well combined.
2. Add the spinach and stir to combine.
3. Divide the spinach mixture into 6 greased cups of an egg bite mold evenly.
4. Press "Power Button" of Ninja Foodi Digital Air Fry Oven and turn the dial to select "Air Fry" mode.
5. Press "Time Button" and again turn the dial to set the cooking time to 17 minutes.
6. Now push "Temp Button" and rotate the dial to set the temperature at 325 degrees F.
7. Press "Start/Pause" button to start.
8. When the unit beeps to show that it is preheated, open the lid.
9. Arrange the mold over the wire rack and insert in the oven.
10. When cooking time is complete, open the lid and place the mold onto a wire rack to cool for about 5 minutes.
11. Top with bacon pieces and serve warm.
12. Serving Suggestions: Serve these muffins with the drizzling of melted butter.
13. Variation Tip: Don't forget to grease the egg bite molds before pacing the egg mixture in them.

Nutrition Info: Calories: 179 Fat: 12.9g Sat Fat: 4.3g Carbohydrates: 1.8g Fiber: 0.1g Sugar: 1.3g Protein: 13.5g

Sausage With Eggs & Avocado

Servings: 2
Cooking Time: 10 Minutes

Ingredients:
- 1 tablespoon maple syrup
- 1 tablespoon balsamic vinegar
- 4 cooked chicken sausages
- 2 hard-boiled eggs, peeled
- 1 small avocado, peeled, pitted and sliced

Directions:
1. In a bowl, mix together the maple syrup and vinegar.
2. Coat the sausages with vinegar mixture.
3. Line the "Sheet Pan" with a lightly, grease piece of foil.
4. Arrange the sausages into the prepared "Sheet Pan".
5. Press "Power Button" of Ninja Foodi Digital Air Fry Oven and turn the dial to select the "Air Roast" mode.
6. Press the Time button and again turn the dial to set the cooking time to 10 minutes.
7. Now push the Temp button and rotate the dial to set the temperature at 450 degrees F.
8. Press "Start/Pause" button to start.
9. When the unit beeps to show that it is preheated, open the lid and insert "Sheet Pan" in the oven.
10. Flip the sausages and coat with the remaining syrup mixture once halfway through.
11. Divide the sausages, eggs and avocado slices onto serving plates and serve.

Nutrition Info: Calories 490 Total Fat 32 g Saturated Fat 8.9 g Cholesterol 164mg Sodium 666 mg Total Carbs 22.1 g Fiber 4.7 g Sugar 7.2 g Protein 26.1 g

French Toast Sticks

Servings: 2
Cooking Time: 10 Minutes

Ingredients:
- 4 slices of thick bread
- 2 eggs, lightly beaten
- 1 teaspoon cinnamon
- 1 teaspoon of vanilla extract
- ¼ cup milk

Directions:
1. Cut the bread into slices for making sticks.
2. Keep parchment paper on the air fryer basket's bottom.
3. Preheat your air fryer to 180 degrees C or 360 degrees F.
4. Now stir together the milk, eggs, cinnamon, vanilla extract, and nutmeg (optional). Combine well.
5. Dip each bread piece into the egg mix. Submerge well.
6. Remove the excess fluid by shaking it well.
7. Keep them in the fryer basket in a single layer.
8. Cook without overcrowding your fryer.

Nutrition Info: Calories 241, Carbohydrates 29g, Cholesterol 188mg, Total Fat 9g, Protein 11g, Fiber 2g, Sodium 423mg, Sugars 4g

Bell Pepper Omelet

Servings: 2
Cooking Time: 10 Minutes

Ingredients:
- 1 teaspoon butter
- 1 small onion, sliced
- ½ of green bell pepper, seeded and chopped
- 4 eggs
- ¼ teaspoon milk
- Salt and ground black pepper, as required
- ¼ cup Cheddar cheese, grated

Directions:
1. In a skillet, melt the butter over medium heat and cook the onion and bell pepper for about 4-5 minutes.
2. Remove the skillet from heat and set aside to cool slightly.
3. Meanwhile, in a bowl, add the eggs, milk, salt and black pepper and beat well.
4. Add the cooked onion mixture and gently, stir to combine.
5. Place the zucchini mixture into a small baking pan.
6. Press "Power Button" of Ninja Foodi Digital Air Fry Oven and turn the dial to select the "Air Fry" mode.
7. Press the Time button and again turn the dial to set the cooking time to 5 minutes.
8. Now push the Temp button and rotate the dial to set the temperature at 355 degrees F.
9. Press "Start/Pause" button to start.
10. When the unit beeps to show that it is preheated, open the lid.
11. Arrange pan over the "Wire Rack" and insert in the oven.
12. Cut the omelet into 2 portions and serve hot.

Nutrition Info: Calories 223 Total Fat 15.5 g Saturated Fat 6.9 g Cholesterol 347 mg Sodium 304 mg Total Carbs 6.4 g Fiber 1.2 g Sugar 3.8 g Protein 15.3 g

Baked Eggs

Servings: 4
Cooking Time: 12 Minutes

Ingredients:
- 1 cup marinara sauce, divided
- 1 tablespoon capers, drained and divided
- 8 eggs
- ¼ cup whipping cream, divided
- ¼ cup Parmesan cheese, shredded and divided
- Salt and ground black pepper, as required

Directions:
1. Grease 4 ramekins. Set aside.
2. Divide the marinara sauce in the bottom of each prepared ramekin evenly and top with capers.
3. Carefully, crack 2 eggs over marinara sauce into each ramekin and top with cream, followed by the Parmesan cheese.
4. Sprinkle each ramekin with salt and black pepper.
5. Press "Power Button" of Ninja Foodi Digital Air Fry Oven and turn the dial to select the "Air Bake" mode.
6. Press the Time button and again turn the dial to set the cooking time to 12 minutes.
7. Now push the Temp button and rotate the dial to set the temperature at 400 degrees F.
8. Press "Start/Pause" button to start.
9. When the unit beeps to show that it is preheated, open the lid.
10. Arrange the ramekins over the "Wire Rack" and insert in the oven.
11. Serve warm.

Nutrition Info: Calories 223 Total Fat 14.1 g Saturated Fat 5.5 g Cholesterol 341 mg Sodium 569 mg Total Carbs 9.8 g Fiber 1.7 g Sugar 6.2 g Protein 14.3 g

Egg & Spinach Tart

Servings: 4
Cooking Time: 25 Minutes

Ingredients:
- 1 puff pastry sheet, trimmed into a 9x13-inch rectangle
- 4 eggs
- ½ cup cheddar cheese, grated
- 7 cooked thick-cut bacon strips
- ½ cup cooked spinach
- 1 egg, lightly beaten

Directions:
1. Arrange the pastry in a lightly greased "Sheet Pan".
2. With a small knife gently, cut a 1-inch border around the edges of the puff pastry without cutting all the way through.
3. With a fork, pierce the center of pastry a few times.
4. Press "Power Button" of Ninja Foodi Digital Air Fry Oven and turn the dial to select the "Air Bake" mode.
5. Press the Time button and again turn the dial to set the cooking time to 10 minutes.
6. Now push the Temp button and rotate the dial to set the temperature at 400 degrees F.
7. Press "Start/Pause" button to start.
8. When the unit beeps to show that it is preheated, open the lid.
9. Insert the "Sheet Pan" in the oven.
10. Remove the "Sheet Pan" from oven and sprinkle the cheese over the center.
11. Place the spinach and bacon in an even layer across the tart.
12. Now, crack the eggs, leaving space between each one.
13. Press "Power Button" of Ninja Foodi Digital Air Fry Oven and turn the dial to select the "Air Bake" mode.
14. Press the Time button and again turn the dial to set the cooking time to 15 minutes.
15. Now push the Temp button and rotate the dial to set the temperature at 400 degrees F.
16. Press "Start/Pause" button to start.
17. When the unit beeps to show that it is preheated, open the lid.
18. Insert the "Sheet Pan" in the oven.
19. Remove the "Sheet Pan" from oven and set aside to cool for 2-3 minutes before cutting.
20. With a pizza cutter, cut into4 portions and serve.

Nutrition Info: Calories 231 Total Fat 17.4 g Saturated Fat 8.2 g Cholesterol 236 mg Sodium 403 mg Total Carbs 5.7 g Fiber 0.3 g Sugar 0.8 g Protein 13.8 g

Tex-mex Hash Browns

Servings: 4
Cooking Time: 30 Minutes

Ingredients:
- 1-1/2 24 oz. potatoes, cut and peeled
- 1 onion, cut into small pieces
- 1 tablespoon of olive oil
- 1 jalapeno, seeded and cut
- 1 red bell pepper, seeded and cut

Directions:
1. Soak the potatoes in water.
2. Preheat your air fryer to 160 degrees C or 320 degrees F.
3. Drain and dry the potatoes using a clean towel.
4. Keep in a bowl.
5. Drizzle some olive oil over the potatoes, coat well.
6. Transfer to the air frying basket.
7. Add the onion, jalapeno, and bell pepper in the bowl.
8. Sprinkle half teaspoon olive oil, pepper, and salt. Coat well by tossing.
9. Now transfer your potatoes to the bowl with the veg mix from your fryer.
10. Place the empty basket into the air fryer. Raise the temperature to 180 degrees C or 356 degrees F.
11. Toss the contents of your bowl for mixing the potatoes with the vegetables evenly.
12. Transfer mix into the basket.
13. Cook until the potatoes have become crispy and brown.

Nutrition Info: Calories 197, Carbohydrates 34g, Cholesterol 0mg, Total Fat 5g, Protein 4g, Fiber 5g, Sodium 79mg, Sugars 3g

Breakfast Frittata

Servings: 2
Cooking Time: 20 Minutes

Ingredients:
- 4 eggs, beaten lightly
- 4 oz. sausages, cooked and crumbled
- 1 onion, chopped
- 2 tablespoons of red bell pepper, diced
- ½ cup shredded Cheddar cheese

Directions:
1. Bring together the cheese, eggs, sausage, onion, and bell pepper in a bowl.
2. Mix well.
3. Preheat your air fryer to 180 degrees C or 360 degrees F.
4. Apply cooking spray lightly.
5. Keep your egg mix in a prepared cake pan.
6. Now cook in your air fryer till the frittata has become set.

Nutrition Info: Calories 487, Carbohydrates 3g, Cholesterol 443mg, Total Fat 39g, Protein 31g, Fiber 0.4g, Sodium 694mg, Sugars 1g

Cheese Toasts With Eggs & Bacon

Servings: 2
Cooking Time: 4 Minutes

Ingredients:
- 4 bread slices
- 1 garlic clove, minced
- 4 ounces goat cheese, crumbled
- Freshly ground black pepper, to taste
- 2 hard-boiled eggs, peeled and chopped
- 4 cooked bacon slices, crumbled

Directions:
1. In a food processor, add the garlic, ricotta, lemon zest and black pepper and pulse until smooth.
2. Spread ricotta mixture over each bread slices evenly.
3. Press "Power Button" of Ninja Foodi Digital Air Fry Oven and turn the dial to select the "Air Fry" mode.
4. Press the Time button and again turn the dial to set the cooking time to 4 minutes.
5. Now push the Temp button and rotate the dial to set the temperature at 355 degrees F.
6. Press "Start/Pause" button to start.
7. When the unit beeps to show that it is preheated, open the lid and lightly, grease the sheet pan.
8. Arrange the bread slices into "Air Fry Basket" and insert in the oven.
9. Top with egg and bacon pieces and serve.

Nutrition Info: Calories 416 Total Fat 29.2 g Saturated Fat 16.9 g Cholesterol 232 mg Sodium 531 mg Total Carbs 11.2 g Fiber 0.5 g Sugar 2.4 g Protein 27.2 g

Banana Bread

Servings: 8
Cooking Time: 45 Minutes

Ingredients:
- ¾ cup whole wheat flour
- 2 medium ripe mashed bananas
- 2 large eggs
- 1 teaspoon of Vanilla extract
- ¼ teaspoon Baking soda
- ½ cup granulated sugar

Directions:
1. Keep parchment paper at the bottom of your pan. Apply some cooking spray.
2. Whisk together the baking soda, salt, flour, and cinnamon (optional) in a bowl.
3. Keep it aside.
4. Take another bowl and bring together the eggs, bananas, vanilla, and yogurt (optional) in it.
5. Stir the wet ingredients gently into your flour mix. Combine well.
6. Now pour your batter into the pan. You can also sprinkle some walnuts.
7. Heat your air fryer to 310°F. Cook till it turns brown.
8. Keep the bread on your wire rack so that it cools in the pan. Slice.

Nutrition Info: Calories 240, Carbohydrates 29g, Total Fat 12g, Protein 4g, Fiber 2g, Sodium 184mg, Sugars 17g

Cinnamon And Sugar Doughnuts

Servings: 9
Cooking Time: 16 Minutes

Ingredients:
- 1 teaspoon cinnamon
- 1/3 cup of white sugar
- 2 large egg yolks
- 2-1/2 tablespoons of butter, room temperature
- 1-1/2 teaspoons baking powder
- 2-1/4 cups of all-purpose flour

Directions:
1. Take a bowl and press your butter and white sugar together in it.
2. Add the egg yolks. Stir till it combines well.
3. Now sift the baking powder, flour, and salt in another bowl.
4. Keep one-third of the flour mix and half of the sour cream into your egg-sugar mixture. Stir till it combines well.
5. Now mix the remaining sour cream and flour. Refrigerate till you can use it.
6. Bring together the cinnamon and one-third sugar in your bowl.
7. Roll half-inch-thick dough.
8. Cut large slices (9) in this dough. Create a small circle in the center. This will make doughnut shapes.
9. Preheat your fryer to 175 degrees C or 350 degrees F.
10. Brush melted butter on both sides of your doughnut.
11. Keep half of the doughnuts in the air fryer's basket.
12. Apply the remaining butter on the cooked doughnuts.
13. Dip into the sugar-cinnamon mix immediately.

Nutrition Info: Calories 336, Carbohydrates 44g, Cholesterol 66mg, Total Fat 16g, Protein 4g, Fiber 1g, Sodium 390mg, Sugars 19g

Roasted Cauliflower

Servings: 2
Cooking Time: 15 Minutes

Ingredients:
- 4 cups of cauliflower florets
- 1 tablespoon peanut oil
- 3 cloves garlic
- ½ teaspoon smoked paprika
- ½ teaspoon of salt

Directions:
1. Preheat your air fryer to 200 degrees C or 400 degrees F.
2. Now cut the garlic into half. Use a knife to smash it.
3. Keep in a bowl with salt, paprika, and oil.
4. Add the cauliflower. Coat well.
5. Transfer the coated cauliflower to your air fryer.
6. Cook for 10 minutes. Shake after 5 minutes.

Nutrition Info: Calories 136, Carbohydrates 12g, Cholesterol 0mg, Total Fat 8g, Protein 4g, Fiber 5.3g, Sodium 642mg, Sugars 5g

Sweet Potato Tots

Servings: 4
Cooking Time: 1 Hour

Ingredients:
- 1 tablespoon of potato starch
- 2 small sweet potatoes, peeled
- 1-1/4 teaspoons kosher salt
- 1/8 teaspoon of garlic powder
- ¾ cup ketchup

Directions:
1. Boil water in a medium-sized pot over high heat.
2. Add the potatoes. Cook till it becomes tender. Transfer them to a plate for cooling. Grate them in a mid-sized bowl.
3. Toss gently with garlic powder, 1 teaspoon of salt, and potato starch.
4. Shape the mix into tot-shaped cylinders.
5. Apply cooking spray on the air fryer basket.
6. Place half of the tots in a later in your basket. Apply some cooking spray.
7. Cook till it becomes light brown at 400°F.
8. Take out from the frying basket. Sprinkle some salt.
9. Serve with ketchup immediately.

Nutrition Info: Calories 80, Carbohydrates 19g, Total Fat 0g, Protein 1g, Fiber 2g, Sodium 335mg, Sugars 8g

Garlic Cheese Bread

Servings: 2
Cooking Time: 10 Minutes

Ingredients:
- 1 cup mozzarella cheese, shredded
- 1 large egg
- ¼ cup parmesan cheese, grated
- ½ teaspoon garlic powder

Directions:
1. Use parchment paper to line your air fryer basket.
2. Bring together the parmesan cheese, mozzarella cheese, garlic powder, and egg in your bowl.
3. Mix until it combines well.
4. Now create a round circle on the parchment paper in your fryer basket.
5. Heat your air fryer to 175 degrees C or 350 degrees F.
6. Fry the bread. Take out and serve warm.

Nutrition Info: Calories 294, Carbohydrates 3g, Cholesterol 138mg, Total Fat 22g, Protein 21g, Fiber 0.1g, Sodium 538mg, Sugars 1g

Potato Rosti

Servings: 2
Cooking Time: 15 Minutes

Ingredients:
- ½ pound potatoes, peeled, grated and squeezed
- ½ tablespoon fresh rosemary, chopped finely
- ½ tablespoon fresh thyme, chopped finely
- 1/8 teaspoon red pepper flakes, crushed
- Salt and ground black pepper, as required
- 2 tablespoons butter, softened

Directions:
1. In a bowl, mix together the potato, herbs, red pepper flakes, salt and black pepper.
2. Press "Power Button" of Ninja Foodi Digital Air Fry Oven and turn the dial to select the "Air Fry" mode.
3. Press the Time button and again turn the dial to set the cooking time to 15 minutes.
4. Now push the Temp button and rotate the dial to set the temperature at 355 degrees F.
5. Press "Start/Pause" button to start.
6. When the unit beeps to show that it is preheated, open the lid and lightly, grease the sheet pan.
7. Arrange the potato mixture into the "Sheet Pan" and shape it into an even circle.
8. Insert the "Sheet Pan" in the oven.
9. Cut the potato rosti into wedges.
10. Top with the butter and serve immediately.

Nutrition Info: Calories 185 Total Fat 11.8 g Saturated Fat 7.4 g Cholesterol 31 mg Sodium 167 mg Total Carbs 18.9 g Fiber 3.4 g Sugar 1.3 g Protein 2.1 g

FISH & SEAFOOD RECIPES

Air Fryer Salmon

Servings: 2
Cooking Time: 6 Minutes

Ingredients:
- 5 oz. filets of salmon
- ¼ cup mayonnaise
- ¼ cup of pistachios, chopped finely
- 1-1/2 tablespoons of minced dill
- 2 tablespoons of lemon juice

Directions:
1. Preheat your air fryer to 400 degrees F.
2. Spray olive oil on the basket.
3. Season your salmon with pepper to taste. You can also apply the all-purpose seasoning.
4. Combine the mayonnaise, lemon juice, and dill in a bowl.
5. Pour a spoonful on the fillets.
6. Top the fillets with chopped pistachios. Be generous.
7. Spray olive oil on the salmon lightly.
8. Air fry your fillets now for 5 minutes.
9. Take out the salmon carefully with a spatula from your air fryer.
10. Keep on a plate. Garnish with dill.

Nutrition Info: Calories 305, Carbohydrates 1g, Cholesterol 43mg, Total Fat 21g, Protein 28g, Fiber 2g, Sugar 3g, Sodium 92mg

Herbed Scallops

Servings: 2
Cooking Time: 14 Minutes

Ingredients:
- ¾ pound sea scallops, cleaned and pat dry
- 1 tablespoon butter, melted
- ¼ tablespoon fresh thyme, minced
- ¼ tablespoon fresh rosemary, minced
- Salt and freshly ground black pepper, to taste

Directions:
1. In a large bowl, place the scallops, butter, herbs, salt, and black pepper and toss to coat well.
2. Press "Power Button" of Ninja Foodi Digital Air Fry Oven and turn the dial to select "Air Fry" mode.
3. Press "Time Button" and again turn the dial to set the cooking time to 4 minutes.
4. Now push "Temp Button" and rotate the dial to set the temperature at 390 degrees F.
5. Press "Start/Pause" button to start.
6. When the unit beeps to show that it is preheated, open the lid and grease the air fry basket.
7. Arrange the scallops into the air fry basket and insert in the oven.
8. When cooking time is complete, open the lid and transfer the scallops onto serving plates.
9. Serve hot.
10. Serving Suggestions: Potato fries will be great with these scallops.
11. Variation Tip: Remove the side muscles from the scallops.

Nutrition Info: Calories: 203 Fat: 7.1g Sat Fat: 3.8g Carbohydrates: 4.5g Fiber: 0.3g Sugar: 0g Protein: 28.7g

Halibut & Shrimp With Pasta

Servings: 4
Cooking Time: 10 Minutes

Ingredients:
- 14 ounces pasta
- 4 tablespoons pesto, divided
- 4 (4-ounce) halibut steaks
- 2 tablespoons olive oil
- ½ pound tomatoes, chopped
- 8 large shrimp, peeled and deveined
- 2 tablespoons fresh lime juice
- 2 tablespoons fresh dill, chopped

Directions:
1. In the bottom of a baking pan, spread 1 tablespoon of pesto.
2. Place halibut steaks and tomatoes over pesto in a single layer and drizzle with the oil.
3. Now, place the shrimp on top in a single layer.
4. Drizzle with lime juice and sprinkle with dill.
5. Press "Power Button" of Ninja Foodi Digital Air Fry Oven and turn the dial to select "Air Fry" mode.
6. Press "Time Button" and again turn the dial to set the cooking time to 8 minutes.
7. Now push "Temp Button" and rotate the dial to set the temperature at 390 degrees F.
8. Press "Start/Pause" button to start.
9. When the unit beeps to show that it is preheated, open the lid.
10. Place the pan over the wire rack and insert in the oven.
11. Meanwhile, in a large pan of salted boiling water, add the pasta and cook for about 8-10 minutes or until desired doneness.
12. Drain the pasta and transfer into a large bowl.
13. Add the remaining pesto and toss to coat well.
14. When cooking time is complete, open the lid and divide the pasta onto serving plates.
15. Top with the fish mixture and serve immediately.
16. Serving Suggestions: Serve with the topping of freshly grated Parmesan.
17. Variation Tip: Linguine pasta will be the best choice for this recipe.

Nutrition Info: Calories: 606 Fat: 19.4g Sat Fat: 3.2g Carbohydrates: 59.1g Fiber: 1.1g Sugar: 2.5g Protein: 47.4g

Spiced Tilapia

Servings: 2
Cooking Time: 12 Minutes

Ingredients:
- ¼ teaspoon garlic powder
- ¼ teaspoon onion powder
- ¼ teaspoon ground cumin
- Salt and ground black pepper, as required
- 2 (6-ounce) tilapia fillets
- 1 tablespoon butter, melted

Directions:
1. In a small bowl, mix together the spices, salt and black pepper.
2. Coat the tilapia fillets with oil and then rub with spice mixture.
3. Press "Power Button" of Ninja Foodi Digital Air Fry Oven and turn the dial to select the "Air Fry" mode.
4. Press the Time button and again turn the dial to set the cooking time to 12 minutes.
5. Now push the Temp button and rotate the dial to set the temperature at 360 degrees F.
6. Press "Start/Pause" button to start.
7. When the unit beeps to show that it is preheated, open the lid.
8. Arrange the tilapia fillets over the greased "Wire Rack" and insert in the oven.
9. Flip the tilapia fillets once halfway through.
10. Serve hot.

Nutrition Info: Calories 194 Total Fat 7.4 g Saturated Fat 4.3 g Cholesterol 98 mg Sodium 179 mg Total Carbs 0.6 g Fiber 0.1 g Sugar 0.2 g Protein 31.8 g

Green Beans With Southern Catfish

Servings: 2
Cooking Time: 10 Minutes

Ingredients:
- 2 catfish fillets
- ¾ oz. green beans, trimmed
- 1 large egg, beaten lightly
- 2 tablespoons of mayonnaise
- 1 teaspoon light brown sugar
- 1/3 cup breadcrumbs
- ½ teaspoon of apple cider vinegar

Directions:
1. Keep the green beans in a bowl. Apply cooking spray liberally.
2. Sprinkle some brown sugar, a pint of salt, and crushed red pepper (optional).
3. Keep in your air fryer basket. Cook at 400 degrees F until it becomes tender and brown.
4. Transfer to your bowl. Use aluminum foil to cover.
5. Toss the catfish in flour. Shake off the excesses.
6. Dip the pieces into the egg. Coat all sides evenly. Sprinkle breadcrumbs.
7. Keep fish in the fryer basket. Apply cooking spray.
8. Now cook at 400 degrees F until it is cooked thoroughly and brown.
9. Sprinkle pepper and ¼ teaspoon of salt.
10. Whisk together the vinegar, sugar, and mayonnaise in a bowl.
11. Serve the fish with tartar sauce and green beans.

Nutrition Info: Calories 562, Carbohydrates 31g, Total Fat 34g, Protein 33g, Fiber 7g, Sugar 16g, Sodium 677mg

Herbed Salmon

Servings: 2
Cooking Time: 10 Minutes

Ingredients:
- 1 tablespoon fresh lime juice
- ½ tablespoons olive oil
- Salt and freshly ground black pepper, to taste
- 1 garlic clove, minced
- ½ teaspoon fresh thyme leaves, chopped
- ½ teaspoon fresh rosemary, chopped
- 2 (7-ounce) salmon fillets

Directions:
1. In a bowl, add all the ingredients except the salmon and mix well.
2. Add the salmon fillets and coat with the mixture generously.
3. Press "Power Button" of Ninja Foodi Digital Air Fry Oven and turn the dial to select "Air Bake" mode.
4. Press "Time Button" and again turn the dial to set the cooking time to 10 minutes.
5. Now push "Temp Button" and rotate the dial to set the temperature at 400 degrees F.
6. Press "Start/Pause" button to start.
7. When the unit beeps to show that it is preheated, open the lid.
8. Arrange the salmon fillets over the greased wire rack and insert in the oven.
9. Flip the fillets once halfway through.
10. When cooking time is complete, open the lid and transfer the salmon fillets onto serving plates.
11. Serve hot.
12. Serving Suggestions: Serve with steamed asparagus.
13. Variation Tip: For best result, use freshly squeezed lime juice.

Nutrition Info: Calories: 297 Fat: 15.8g Sat Fat: 2.3g Carbohydrates: 0.9g Fiber: 0.3g Sugar: 0g Protein: 38.6g

Grilled Fish Fillet In Pesto Sauce

Servings: 2
Cooking Time: 8 Minutes

Ingredients:
- 2 fish fillets, white fish
- 1 tablespoon of olive oil
- 2 cloves of garlic
- 1 bunch basil
- 1 tablespoon Parmesan cheese, grated

Directions:
1. Heat your air fryer to 180 degrees C.
2. Brush oil on your fish fillets. Season with salt and pepper.
3. Keep in your basket and into the fryer.
4. Cook for 6 minutes.
5. Keep the basil leaves with the cheese, olive oil, and garlic in your food processor.
6. Pulse until it becomes a sauce. Include salt to taste.
7. Keep fillets on your serving plate. Serve with pesto sauce.

Nutrition Info: Calories 1453, Carbohydrates 3g, Cholesterol 58mg, Total Fat 141g, Protein 43g, Fiber 1g, Sugar 0g, Sodium 1773mg

Prawn Burgers

Servings: 2
Cooking Time: 6 Minutes

Ingredients:
- ½ cup prawns, peeled, deveined and chopped very finely
- ½ cup breadcrumbs
- 2-3 tablespoons onion, chopped finely
- ½ teaspoon fresh ginger, minced
- ½ teaspoon garlic, minced
- ½ teaspoon red chili powder
- ½ teaspoon ground cumin
- ¼ teaspoon ground turmeric
- Salt and freshly ground black pepper, to taste

Directions:
1. In a bowl, add all ingredients and mix until well combined.
2. Make small sized patties from mixture.
3. Press "Power Button" of Ninja Foodi Digital Air Fry Oven and turn the dial to select "Air Fry" mode.
4. Press "Time Button" and again turn the dial to set the cooking time to 6 minutes.
5. Now push "Temp Button" and rotate the dial to set the temperature at 355 degrees F.
6. Press "Start/Pause" button to start.
7. When the unit beeps to show that it is preheated, open the lid and grease the air fry basket.
8. Arrange the patties into the prepared air fry basket and insert in the oven.
9. When cooking time is complete, open the lid and transfer the burgers onto serving plates.
10. Serve hot.
11. Serving Suggestions: Serve with tomato ketchup.
12. Variation Tip: Don't use frozen shrimp in this recipe.

Nutrition Info: Calories: 186 Fat: 2.7g Sat Fat: 0.7g Carbohydrates: 22.5g Fiber: 1.8g Sugar: 2.2g Protein: 16.9g

Zesty Fish Fillets

Servings: 4
Cooking Time: 12 Minutes

Ingredients:
- 4 fillets of salmon or tilapia
- 2-1/2 teaspoons vegetable oil
- ¾ cups crushed cornflakes or bread crumbs
- 2 eggs, beaten
- 1 packet dry dressing mix

Directions:
1. Preheat the air fryer to 180° C.
2. Mix the dressing mix and the breadcrumbs together.
3. Pour the oil. Stir until you see the mix getting crumbly and loose.
4. Now dip your fish fillets into the egg. Remove the excess.
5. Dip your fillets into the crumb mix. Coat evenly.
6. Transfer to the fryer carefully.
7. Cook for 10 minutes. Take out and serve.
8. You can also add some lemon wedges on your fish.

Nutrition Info: Calories 382, Carbohydrates 8g, Cholesterol 166mg, Total Fat 22g, Protein 38g, Sodium 220mg, Calcium 50mg

Crusted Sole

Servings: 2
Cooking Time: 15 Minutes

Ingredients:
- 2 teaspoons mayonnaise
- 1 teaspoon fresh chives, minced
- 3 tablespoons Parmesan cheese, shredded
- 2 tablespoons panko breadcrumbs
- Salt and freshly ground black pepper, to taste
- 2 (4-ounce) sole fillets

Directions:
1. In a shallow dish, mix together the mayonnaise and chives.
2. In another shallow dish, mix together the cheese, breadcrumbs, salt and black pepper.
3. Coat the fish fillets with mayonnaise mixture and then roll in cheese mixture.
4. Arrange the sole fillets onto the greased sheet pan in a single layer.
5. Press "Power Button" of Ninja Foodi Digital Air Fry Oven and turn the dial to select "Air Bake" mode.
6. Press "Time Button" and again turn the dial to set the cooking time to 15 minutes.
7. Now push "Temp Button" and rotate the dial to set the temperature at 450 degrees F.
8. Press "Start/Pause" button to start.
9. When the unit beeps to show that it is preheated, open the lid and insert the sheet pan in the oven.
10. When cooking time is complete, open the lid and transfer the fish fillets onto serving plates.
11. Serve hot.
12. Serving Suggestions: Roasted potatoes make a great side for fish.
13. Variation Tip: If you want a gluten-free option then use pork rinds instead of breadcrumbs.

Nutrition Info: Calories: 584 Fat: 14.6g Sat Fat: 5.2g Carbohydrates: 16.7g Fiber: 0.4g Sugar: 0.2g Protein: 33.2g

Crusted Salmon

Servings: 2
Cooking Time: 15 Minutes

Ingredients:
- 2 (6-ounce) skinless salmon fillets
- Salt and ground black pepper, as required
- 3 tablespoons walnuts, chopped finely
- 3 tablespoons quick-cooking oats, crushed
- 2 tablespoons olive oil

Directions:
1. Rub the salmon fillets with salt and black pepper evenly.
2. In a bowl, mix together the walnuts, oats and oil.
3. Arrange the salmon fillets onto the greased "Sheet Pan" in a single layer.
4. Place the oat mixture over salmon fillets and gently, press down.
5. Press "Power Button" of Ninja Foodi Digital Air Fry Oven and turn the dial to select the "Air Bake" mode.
6. Press the Time button and again turn the dial to set the cooking time to 15 minutes.
7. Now push the Temp button and rotate the dial to set the temperature at 400 degrees F.
8. Press "Start/Pause" button to start.
9. When the unit beeps to show that it is preheated, open the lid.
10. Insert the "Sheet Pan" in oven.
11. Serve hot.

Nutrition Info: Calories 446 Total Fat 31.9 g Saturated Fat 4 g Cholesterol 75 mg Sodium 153 mg Total Carbs 6.4 g Fiber 1.6 g Sugar 0.2 g Protein 36.8 g

Pesto Salmon

Servings: 4
Cooking Time: 15 Minutes

Ingredients:
- 1¼ pound salmon fillet, cut into 4 fillets
- 2 tablespoons white wine
- 1 tablespoon fresh lemon juice
- 2 tablespoons pesto, thawed
- 2 tablespoons pine nuts, toasted

Directions:
1. Arrange the salmon fillets onto q foil-lined baking pan, skin-side down.
2. Drizzle the salmon fillets with wine and lemon juice.
3. Set aside for about 15 minutes.
4. Spread pesto over each salmon fillet evenly.
5. Press "Power Button" of Ninja Foodi Digital Air Fry Oven and turn the dial to select the "Air Broil" mode.
6. Press the Time button and again turn the dial to set the cooking time to 15 minutes.
7. Press "Start/Pause" button to start.
8. When the unit beeps to show that it is preheated, open the lid.
9. Insert the baking pan in oven.
10. Garnish with toasted pine nuts and serve.

Nutrition Info: Calories 257 Total Fat 15 g Saturated Fat 2.1 g Cholesterol 64 mg Sodium 111 mg Total Carbs 1.3 g Fiber 0.3 g Sugar 0.8 g Protein 28.9 g

Seasoned Catfish

Servings: 4
Cooking Time: 23 Minutes

Ingredients:
- 4 (4-ounce) catfish fillets
- 2 tablespoons Italian seasoning
- Salt and freshly ground black pepper, to taste
- 1 tablespoon olive oil
- 1 tablespoon fresh parsley, chopped

Directions:
1. Rub the fish fillets with seasoning, salt and black pepper generously and then coat with oil.
2. Press "Power Button" of Ninja Foodi Digital Air Fry Oven and turn the dial to select "Air Fry" mode.
3. Press "Time Button" and again turn the dial to set the cooking time to 20 minutes.
4. Now push "Temp Button" and rotate the dial to set the temperature at 400 degrees F.
5. Press "Start/Pause" button to start.
6. When the unit beeps to show that it is preheated, open the lid and grease the air fry basket.
7. Arrange the fish fillets into the prepared air fry basket and insert in the oven.
8. Flip the fish fillets once halfway through.
9. When cooking time is complete, open the lid and transfer the fillets onto serving plates.
10. Serve hot with the garnishing of parsley.
11. Serving Suggestions: Quinoa salad will be a great choice for serving.
12. Variation Tip: Season the fish according to your choice.

Nutrition Info: Calories: 205 Fat: 14.2g Sat Fat: 2.4g Carbohydrates: 0.8g Fiber: 0g Sugar: 0.6g Protein: 17.7g

Crumbed Fish

Servings: 4
Cooking Time: 12 Minutes

Ingredients:
- 4 flounder fillets
- 1 cup bread crumbs
- 1 egg, beaten
- ¼ cup of vegetable oil
- 1 lemon, sliced

Directions:
1. Preheat your air fryer to 180 degrees C or 350 degrees F.
2. Mix the oil and bread crumbs in a bowl. Keep stirring until you see this mixture becoming crumbly and loose.
3. Now dip your fish fillets into the egg. Remove any excess.
4. Dip your fillets into the bread crumb mix. Make sure to coat evenly.
5. Keep the coated fillets in your preheated fryer gently.
6. Cook until you see the fish flaking easily with a fork.
7. Add lemon slices for garnishing.

Nutrition Info: Calories 389, Carbohydrates 23g, Cholesterol 107mg, Total Fat 21g, Protein 27g, Fiber 3g, Sodium 309mg, Sugars 2g

Lemon Dill Mahi Mahi

Servings: 2
Cooking Time: 15 Minutes

Ingredients:
- 2 fillets of Mahi Mahi, thawed
- 2 lemon slices
- 1 tablespoon olive oil
- 1 tablespoon lemon juice
- 1 tablespoon dill, chopped

Directions:
1. Combine the olive oil and lemon juice in a bowl. Stir.
2. Keep the fish fillets on a parchment paper sheet.
3. Brush the lemon juice mix on each side. Coat heavily.
4. Season with pepper and salt.
5. Add the chopped dill on top.
6. Keep the fillets of Mahi Mahi in your air fryer basket.
7. Cook at 400° F for 12 minutes.
8. Take out. Serve immediately.

Nutrition Info: Calories 95, Carbohydrates 2g, Cholesterol 21mg, Total Fat 7g, Protein 6g, Sugar 0.2g, Sodium 319mg

Glazed Salmon

Servings: 2
Cooking Time: 8 Minutes

Ingredients:
- 2 (6-ounce) salmon fillets
- Salt, to taste
- 2 tablespoons honey

Directions:
1. Sprinkle the salmon fillets with salt and then coat with honey.
2. Press "Power Button" of Ninja Foodi Digital Air Fry Oven and turn the dial to select "Air Fry" mode.
3. Press "Time Button" and again turn the dial to set the cooking time to 8 minutes.
4. Now push "Temp Button" and rotate the dial to set the temperature at 355 degrees F.
5. Press "Start/Pause" button to start.
6. When the unit beeps to show that it is preheated, open the lid and grease the air fry basket.
7. Arrange the salmon fillets into the prepared air fry basket and insert in the oven.
8. When cooking time is complete, open the lid and transfer the salmon fillets onto serving plates.
9. Serve hot.
10. Serving Suggestions: Fresh baby greens will be great if served with glazed salmon.
11. Variation Tip: honey can be replaced with maple syrup too.

Nutrition Info: Calories: 289 Fat: 10.5g Sat Fat: 1.5g Carbohydrates: 17.3g Fiber: 0g Sugar: 17.3g Protein: 33.1g

Cod Parcel

Servings: 2
Cooking Time: 15 Minutes

Ingredients:
- 2 tablespoons butter, melted
- 1 tablespoon fresh lemon juice
- ½ teaspoon dried tarragon
- Salt and freshly ground black pepper, to taste
- ½ cup red bell peppers, seeded and thinly sliced
- ½ cup carrots, peeled and julienned
- ½ cup fennel bulbs, julienned
- 2 (5-ounce) frozen cod fillets, thawed
- 1 tablespoon olive oil

Directions:
1. In a large bowl, mix together the butter, lemon juice, tarragon, salt, and black pepper.
2. Add the bell pepper, carrot, and fennel bulb and generously coat with the mixture.
3. Arrange 2 large parchment squares onto a smooth surface.
4. Coat the cod fillets with oil and then sprinkle evenly with salt and black pepper.
5. Arrange 1 cod fillet onto each parchment square and top each evenly with the vegetables.
6. Top with any remaining sauce from the bowl.
7. Fold the parchment paper and crimp the sides to secure fish and vegetables.
8. Press "Power Button" of Ninja Foodi Digital Air Fry Oven and turn the dial to select "Air Fry" mode.
9. Press "Time Button" and again turn the dial to set the cooking time to 15 minutes.
10. Now push "Temp Button" and rotate the dial to set the temperature at 350 degrees F.
11. Press "Start/Pause" button to start.
12. When the unit beeps to show that it is preheated, open the lid.
13. Arrange the cod parcels into the air fry basket and insert in the oven.
14. When cooking time is complete, open the lid and transfer the cod parcels onto serving plates.
15. Carefully open the parcels and serve hot.
16. Serving Suggestions: Serve with the drizzling of lime juice.
17. Variation Tip: You can use veggies of your choice.

Nutrition Info: Calories: 306 Fat: 20g Sat Fat: 8.4g Carbohydrates: 6.8g Fiber: 1.8g Sugar: 3g Protein: 26.3g

Ranch Tilapia

Servings: 4
Cooking Time: 13 Minutes

Ingredients:
- ¾ cup cornflakes, crushed
- 1 (1-ounce) packet dry ranch-style dressing mix
- 2½ tablespoons vegetable oil
- 2 eggs
- 4 (6-ounce) tilapia fillets

Directions:
1. In a shallow bowl, crack the eggs and beat slightly.
2. In another bowl, add the cornflakes, ranch dressing, and oil and mix until a crumbly mixture forms.
3. Dip the fish fillets into egg and then, coat with the breadcrumbs mixture.
4. Press "Power Button" of Ninja Foodi Digital Air Fry Oven and turn the dial to select "Air Fry" mode.
5. Press "Time Button" and again turn the dial to set the cooking time to 13 minutes.
6. Now push "Temp Button" and rotate the dial to set the temperature at 356 degrees F.
7. Press "Start/Pause" button to start.
8. When the unit beeps to show that it is preheated, open the lid and grease the air fry basket.
9. Arrange the tilapia fillets into the prepared air fry basket and insert in the oven. When cooking time is complete, open the lid and transfer the fillets onto serving plates.
10. Serve hot.
11. Serving Suggestions: Serve tilapia with lemon butter.
12. Variation Tip: The skin should be removed, either before cooking or before serving.

Nutrition Info: Calories: 267 Fat: 12.2g Sat Fat: 3g Carbohydrates: 5.1g Fiber: 0.2g Sugar: 0.9g Protein: 34.9g

POULTRY RECIPES

Spicy Chicken Legs

Servings: 6
Cooking Time: 25 Minutes
Ingredients:
- 2½ pounds chicken legs
- 2 tablespoons olive oil
- 1 teaspoon smoked paprika
- 1 teaspoon garlic powder
- ½ teaspoon ground cumin
- Salt and freshly ground black pepper, to taste

Directions:
1. In a large bowl, add all the ingredients and mix well.
2. Arrange the chicken legs onto a sheet pan.
3. Press "Power Button" of Ninja Foodi Digital Air Fry Oven and turn the dial to select "Air Fry" mode.
4. Press "Time Button" and again turn the dial to set the cooking time to 25 minutes.
5. Now push "Temp Button" and rotate the dial to set the temperature at 400 degrees F.
6. Press "Start/Pause" button to start.
7. When the unit beeps to show that it is preheated, open the lid and insert the sheet pan in the oven.
8. When cooking time is complete, open the lid and transfer the chicken legs onto serving plates.
9. Serve hot.
10. Serving Suggestions: Serve with cheesy baked asparagus.
11. Variation Tip: Don't accept any chicken legs that are soft and discolored.

Nutrition Info: Calories: 402 Fat: 18.8g Sat Fat: 4.5g Carbohydrates: 0.6g Fiber: 0.2g Sugar: 0.2g Protein: 54.8g

Herbed Turkey Breast

Servings: 6
Cooking Time: 40 Minutes

Ingredients:
- ¼ cup unsalted butter, softened
- 2 tablespoons fresh rosemary, chopped
- 2 tablespoon fresh thyme, chopped
- 2 tablespoons fresh sage, chopped
- 2 tablespoons fresh parsley, chopped
- Salt and freshly ground black pepper, to taste
- 1 (4-pound) bone-in, skin-on turkey breast
- 2 tablespoons olive oil

Directions:
1. In a bowl, add the butter, herbs, salt and black pepper and mix well.
2. Rub the herb mixture under skin evenly.
3. Coat the outside of turkey breast with oil.
4. Place the turkey breast into the greased baking pan.
5. Press "Power Button" of Ninja Foodi Digital Air Fry Oven and turn the dial to select "Air Bake" mode.
6. Press "Time Button" and again turn the dial to set the cooking time to 40 minutes.
7. Now push "Temp Button" and rotate the dial to set the temperature at 350 degrees F.
8. Press "Start/Pause" button to start.
9. When the unit beeps to show that it is preheated, open the lid and insert baking pan in the oven.
10. When cooking time is complete, open the lid and place the turkey breast onto a platter for about 5-10 minutes before slicing.
11. With a sharp knife, cut the turkey breast into desired sized slices and serve.
12. Serving Suggestions: Roasted potatoes will accompany this turkey breast nicely.
13. Variation Tip: Use unsalted butter.

Nutrition Info: Calories: 333 Fat: 37g Sat Fat: 12.4g Carbohydrates: 1.8g Fiber: 1.1g Sugar: 0.1g Protein: 65.1g

Popcorn Chicken

Servings: 4
Cooking Time: 10 Minutes

Ingredients:
- 1 oz. chicken breast halves, boneless and skinless
- ½ teaspoon paprika
- ¼ teaspoon mustard, ground
- ¼ teaspoon of garlic powder
- 3 tablespoons of cornstarch

Directions:
1. Cut the chicken into small pieces and keep in a bowl.
2. Combine the paprika, garlic powder, mustard, salt, and pepper in another bowl.
3. Reserve a teaspoon of your seasoning mixture. Sprinkle the other portion on the chicken. Coat evenly by tossing.
4. Combine the reserved seasoning and cornstarch in a plastic bag.
5. Combine well by shaking.
6. Keep your chicken pieces in the bag. Seal it and shake for coating evenly.
7. Now transfer the chicken to a mesh strainer. Shake the excess cornstarch.
8. Keep aside for 5-10 minutes. The cornstarch should start to get absorbed into your chicken.
9. Preheat your air fryer to 200 degrees C or 390 degrees F.
10. Apply some oil on the air fryer basket.
11. Keep the chicken pieces inside. They should not overlap.
12. Apply cooking spray.
13. Cook until the chicken isn't pink anymore.

Nutrition Info: Calories 156, Carbohydrates 6g, Cholesterol 65mg, Total Fat 4g, Protein 24g, Sugar 0g, Fiber 0.3g, Sodium 493mg

Bang-bang Chicken

Servings: 6
Cooking Time: 15 Minutes

Ingredients:
- 1 oz. chicken breast tenderloins, small pieces
- ½ cup sweet chili sauce
- 1 cup of mayonnaise
- 1-1/2 cups bread crumbs
- 1/3 cup flour

Directions:
1. Whisk the sweet chili sauce and mayonnaise together in a bowl.
2. Spoon out 3 quarters of a cup from this. Set aside.
3. Keep flour in a plastic bag. Add the chicken and close this bag. Coat well by shaking.
4. Place the coated chicken in a large bowl with the mayonnaise mix.
5. Combine well by stirring.
6. Keep your bread crumbs in another plastic bag.
7. Place chicken pieces into the bread crumbs. Coat well.
8. Preheat your air fryer to 200 degrees C or 400 degrees F.
9. Transfer the chicken into the basket of your air fryer. Do not overcrowd.
10. Cook for 7 minutes.
11. Flip over and cook for another 4 minutes.
12. Transfer the chicken to a bowl. Pour over the reserved sauce.
13. You can also sprinkle some green onions before serving.

Nutrition Info: Calories 566, Carbohydrates 35g, Cholesterol 60mg, Total Fat 38g, Protein 21g, Sugar 7g, Fiber 1g, Sodium 818mg

Asian Deviled Eggs

Servings: 12
Cooking Time: 15 Minutes

Ingredients:
- 6 eggs
- 2 tablespoons of mayonnaise
- 1 teaspoon soy sauce, low-sodium
- 1-1/2 teaspoons of sesame oil
- 1 teaspoon Dijon mustard

Directions:
1. Keep the eggs on the air fryer rack. Make sure that there is adequate space between them.
2. Set the temperature to 125 degrees C or 160 degrees F.
3. Air fry for 15 minutes.
4. Take out the eggs from your air fryer. Keep in an ice water bowl for 10 minutes.
5. Take them out of the water. Now peel and cut them in half.
6. Scoop out the yolks carefully. Keep in a food processor.
7. Add the sesame oil, mayonnaise, Dijon mustard, and soy sauce.
8. Process until everything combines well. The mixture should be creamy.
9. Fill up your piping bag with this yolk mixture. Distribute evenly into the egg whites. They should be heaping full.
10. You can garnish with green onions and sesame seeds (optional).

Nutrition Info: Calories 70, Carbohydrates 1g, Cholesterol 94mg, Total Fat 6g, Protein 3g, Sugar 0g, Fiber 0.1g, Sodium 102mg

Roasted Cornish Game Hen

Servings: 4
Cooking Time: 16 Minutes

Ingredients:
- ¼ cup olive oil
- 1 teaspoon fresh rosemary, chopped
- 1 teaspoon fresh thyme, chopped
- 1 teaspoon fresh lemon zest, finely grated
- ¼ teaspoon sugar
- ¼ teaspoon red pepper flakes, crushed
- Salt and freshly ground black pepper, to taste
- 2 pounds Cornish game hen, backbone removed and halved

Directions:
1. In a bowl, mix together oil, herbs, lemon zest, sugar, and spices.
2. Add the hen portions and coat with the marinade generously.
3. Cover and refrigerate for about 24 hours.
4. In a strainer, place the hen portions and set aside to drain any liquid.
5. Press "Power Button" of Ninja Foodi Digital Air Fry Oven and turn the dial to select "Air Fry" mode.
6. Press "Time Button" and again turn the dial to set the cooking time to 16 minutes.
7. Now push "Temp Button" and rotate the dial to set the temperature at 390 degrees F.
8. Press "Start/Pause" button to start.
9. When the unit beeps to show that it is preheated, open the lid and grease the air fry basket.
10. Arrange the hen portions into the prepared basket and insert in the oven.
11. When cooking time is complete, open the lid and transfer the hen portions onto a platter.
12. Cut each portion in half and serve.
13. Serving Suggestions: Serve with dinner rolls.
14. Variation Tip: Place the hens in the basket, breast side up.

Nutrition Info: Calories: 557 Fat: 45.1g Sat Fat: 1.8g Carbohydrates: 0.8g Fiber: 0.3g Sugar: 0.3g Protein: 38.5g

Seasoned Chicken Tenders

Servings: 2
Cooking Time: 10 Minutes

Ingredients:

- 8 ounces chicken tenders
- 1 teaspoon BBQ seasoning
- Salt and ground black pepper, as required

Directions:

1. Line the "Sheet Pan" with a lightly, greased piece of foil.
2. Set aside.
3. Season the chicken tenders with BBQ seasoning, salt and black pepper.
4. Arrange the chicken tenders onto the prepared "Sheet Pan" in a single layer.
5. Press "Power Button" of Ninja Foodi Digital Air Fry Oven and turn the dial to select the "Air Bake" mode.
6. Press the Time button and again turn the dial to set the cooking time to 10 minutes.
7. Now push the Temp button and rotate the dial to set the temperature at 450 degrees F.
8. Press "Start/Pause" button to start.
9. When the unit beeps to show that it is preheated, open the lid and insert "Sheet Pan" in the oven.
10. Serve hot.

Nutrition Info: Calories 220 Total Fat 8.4 g Saturated Fat 2.3 g Cholesterol 101 mg Sodium 315 mg Total Carbs 0.5 g Fiber 0 g Sugar 0 g Protein 32.8 g

Herbed & Spiced Turkey Breast

Servings: 6
Cooking Time: 40 Minutes

Ingredients:
- ¼ cup butter, softened
- 2 tablespoons fresh rosemary, chopped
- 2 tablespoon fresh thyme, chopped
- 2 tablespoons fresh sage, chopped
- 2 tablespoons fresh parsley, chopped
- Salt and ground black pepper, as required
- 1 (4-pound) bone-in, skin-on turkey breast
- 2 tablespoons olive oil

Directions:
1. In a bowl, add the butter, herbs, salt and black pepper and mix well.
2. Rub the herb mixture under skin evenly.
3. Coat the outside of turkey breast with oil.
4. Place the turkey breast into the greased baking pan.
5. Press "Power Button" of Ninja Foodi Digital Air Fry Oven and turn the dial to select the "Air Bake" mode.
6. Press the Time button and again turn the dial to set the cooking time to 40 minutes.
7. Now push the Temp button and rotate the dial to set the temperature at 350 degrees F.
8. Press "Start/Pause" button to start.
9. When the unit beeps to show that it is preheated, open the lid and insert baking pan in the oven.
10. Remove from oven and place the turkey breast onto a platter for about 5-10 minutes before slicing.
11. With a sharp knife, cut the turkey breast into desired sized slices and serve.

Nutrition Info: Calories 333 Total Fat 37 g Saturated Fat 12.4 g Cholesterol 209 mg Sodium 245 mg Total Carbs 1.8 g Fiber 1.1 g Sugar 0.1 g Protein 65.1 g

Hard-boiled Eggs

Servings: 6
Cooking Time: 16 Minutes
Ingredients:
- 6 eggs, large

Directions:
1. Keep the eggs on your air fryer's wire rack.
2. Set the temperature to 250.
3. Take out the eggs once they are done.
4. Place them in a bowl with ice water.
5. Peel them off and serve.

Nutrition Info: Calories 91, Carbohydrates 1g, Total Fat 7g, Protein 6g, Sugar 0g, Fiber 0g, Sodium 62mg

Blackened Chicken Breast

Servings: 2
Cooking Time: 20 Minutes

Ingredients:
- 2 chicken breast halves, skinless and boneless
- 1 teaspoon thyme, ground
- 2 teaspoons of paprika
- 2 teaspoons vegetable oil
- ½ teaspoon onion powder

Directions:
1. Combine the thyme, paprika, onion powder, and salt together in your bowl.
2. Transfer the spice mix to a flat plate.
3. Rub vegetable oil on the chicken breast. Coat fully.
4. Roll the chicken pieces in the spice mixture. Press down, ensuring that all sides have the spice mix.
5. Keep aside for 5 minutes.
6. In the meantime, preheat your air fryer to 175 degrees C or 360 degrees F.
7. Keep the chicken in the air fryer basket. Cook for 8 minutes.
8. Flip once and cook for another 7 minutes.
9. Transfer the breasts to a serving plate. Serve after 5 minutes.

Nutrition Info: Calories 427, Carbohydrates 3g, Cholesterol 198mg, Total Fat 11g, Protein 79g, Sugar 1g, Fiber 2g, Sodium 516mg

Spiced Chicken Thighs

Servings: 4
Cooking Time: 20 Minutes

Ingredients:
- 1 teaspoon ground cumin
- 1 teaspoon garlic powder
- ½ teaspoon smoked paprika
- ½ teaspoon ground coriander
- Salt and ground black pepper, as required
- 4 (5-ounce) chicken thighs

Directions:
1. In a large bowl, add the spices, salt and black pepper and mix well.
2. Coat the chicken thighs with oil and then rub with spice mixture.
3. Arrange the chicken thighs onto the sheet pan.
4. Press "Power Button" of Ninja Foodi Digital Air Fry Oven and turn the dial to select "Air Fry" mode.
5. Press "Time Button" and again turn the dial to set the cooking time to 20 minutes.
6. Now push "Temp Button" and rotate the dial to set the temperature at 400 degrees F.
7. Press "Start/Pause" button to start.
8. When the unit beeps to show that it is preheated, open the lid and insert the sheet pan in the oven.
9. Flip the chicken thighs once halfway through.
10. When cooking time is complete, open the lid and transfer the chicken thighs onto serving plates.
11. Serve hot.
12. Serving Suggestions: Serve with a fresh green salad.
13. Variation Tip: Adjust the ratio of spices according to your spice tolerance.

Nutrition Info: Calories: 334 Fat: 17.7g Sat Fat: 3.9g Carbohydrates: 0.9g Fiber: 0.2g Sugar: 0.2g Protein: 41.3g

Lemony Turkey Legs

Servings: 2
Cooking Time: 30 Minutes

Ingredients:
- 2 garlic cloves, minced
- 1 tablespoon fresh rosemary, minced
- 1 teaspoon fresh lemon zest, finely grated
- 2 tablespoons olive oil
- 1 tablespoon fresh lemon juice
- Salt and freshly ground black pepper, to taste
- 2 turkey legs

Directions:
1. In a large bowl, mix together the garlic, rosemary, lime zest, oil, lime juice, salt, and black pepper.
2. Add the turkey legs and coat with marinade generously.
3. Refrigerate to marinate for about 6-8 hours.
4. Press "Power Button" of Ninja Foodi Digital Air Fry Oven and turn the dial to select "Air Fry" mode.
5. Press "Time Button" and again turn the dial to set the cooking time to 30 minutes.
6. Now push "Temp Button" and rotate the dial to set the temperature at 350 degrees F.
7. Press "Start/Pause" button to start.
8. When the unit beeps to show that it is preheated, open the lid and grease the air fry basket.
9. Arrange the turkey legs into the prepared basket and insert in the oven.
10. Flip the turkey legs once halfway through.
11. When cooking time is complete, open the lid and transfer the turkey legs onto serving plates.
12. Serve hot.
13. Serving Suggestions: Serve these turkey legs with honey macadamia stuffing.
14. Variation Tip: A fresh turkey meat should never be chilled below 26 degrees.

Nutrition Info: Calories: 709 Fat: 32.7g Sat Fat: 7.8g Carbohydrates: 2.3g Fiber: 0.8g Sugar: 0.1g Protein: 97.2g

Air Fryer Chicken Wings

Servings: 4
Cooking Time: 30 Minutes

Ingredients:
- 1-1/2 oz. chicken wings
- 1 teaspoon garlic powder
- 1 teaspoon kosher salt
- 1 tablespoon of butter, unsalted and melted
- ½ cup hot sauce

Directions:
1. Keep your chicken wings in 1 layer. Use paper towels to pat them dry.
2. Sprinkle garlic powder and salt evenly.
3. Now keep these wings in your air fryer at 380°F.
4. Cook for 20 minutes. Toss after every 5 minutes. The wings should be cooked through and tender.
5. Bring up the temperature to 400 degrees F.
6. Cook for 5-8 minutes until it has turned golden brown and crispy.
7. Toss your wings with melted butter (optional) before serving.

Nutrition Info: Calories 291, Carbohydrates 1g, Total Fat 23g, Protein 20g, Sugar 0.3g, Fiber 0g, Sodium 593mg

Thyme Duck Breast

Servings: 2
Cooking Time: 20 Minutes

Ingredients:
- 1 cup beer
- 1 tablespoon olive oil
- 1 teaspoon mustard
- 1 tablespoon fresh thyme, chopped
- Salt and freshly ground black pepper, to taste
- 1 (10½-ounce) duck breast

Directions:
1. In a bowl, add the beer, oil, mustard, thyme, salt, and black pepper and mix well
2. Add the duck breast and coat with marinade generously.
3. Cover and refrigerate for about 4 hours.
4. Arrange the duck breast onto the greased sheet pan.
5. Press "Power Button" of Ninja Foodi Digital Air Fry Oven and turn the dial to select "Air Fry" mode.
6. Press "Time Button" and again turn the dial to set the cooking time to 20 minutes.
7. Now push "Temp Button" and rotate the dial to set the temperature at 390 degrees F.
8. Press "Start/Pause" button to start.
9. When the unit beeps to show that it is preheated, open the lid and insert the sheet pan in the oven.
10. Flip the duck breast once halfway through.
11. When cooking time is complete, open the lid and place the duck breast onto a cutting board for about 5 minutes before slicing.
12. With a sharp knife, cut the duck breast into desired size slices and serve.
13. Serving Suggestions: Duck meat goes really well with caramelized onions or balsamic reduction.
14. Variation Tip: Look for a plump, firm breast for best flav

Nutrition Info: Calories: 315 Fat: 13.5g Sat Fat: 1.1g Carbohydrates: 5.7g Fiber: 0.7g Sugar: 0.1g Protein: 33.8g

Turkish Chicken Kebab

Servings: 4
Cooking Time: 15 Minutes

Ingredients:
- 1 oz. Chicken thighs, boneless and skinless
- ¼ cup Greek yogurt, plain
- 1 tablespoon tomato paste
- 1 tablespoon vegetable oil
- ½ teaspoon cinnamon, ground

Directions:
1. Stir together the tomato paste, Greek yogurt, oil, cinnamon, salt, and pepper in a bowl. The spices should blend well into the yogurt.
2. Cut the chicken into 4 pieces.
3. Now include your chicken pieces into the mixture. Make sure that the chicken is coated well with the mixture.
4. Refrigerate for 30 minutes' minimum.
5. Take out chicken from your marinade.
6. Keep in your air fryer basket in a single layer.
7. Set your fryer to 370 degrees F. Cook the chicken pieces for 8 minutes.
8. Flip over and cook for another 4 minutes.

Nutrition Info: Calories 375, Carbohydrates 4g, Cholesterol 112mg, Total Fat 31g, Protein 20g, Sugar 1g, Fiber 1g

Herbed Roasted Chicken

Servings: 6
Cooking Time: 1 Hour 10 Minutes

Ingredients:
- ¼ cup butter, softened
- 1 teaspoon dried rosemary, crushed
- 1 teaspoon dried basil, crushed
- 1 teaspoon dried oregano, crushed
- 1 teaspoon dried thyme, crushed
- 1 tablespoon garlic powder
- 1 tablespoon paprika
- 1 tablespoon ground cumin
- Salt and freshly ground black pepper, to taste
- 1 (3-pound) whole chicken, neck and giblets removed

Directions:
1. In a bowl, add the butter, herbs, spices and salt and mix well.
2. Rub the chicken with spice mixture generously.
3. With kitchen twine, tie off wings and legs.
4. Arrange the chicken onto the greased sheet pan.
5. Press "Power Button" of Ninja Foodi Digital Air Fry Oven and turn the dial to select "Air Bake" mode.
6. Press "Time Button" and again turn the dial to set the cooking time to 70 minutes.
7. Now push "Temp Button" and rotate the dial to set the temperature at 380 degrees F.
8. Press "Start/Pause" button to start.
9. When the unit beeps to show that it is preheated, open the lid and insert the sheet pan in oven.
10. When cooking time is complete, open the lid and place the chicken onto a platter for about 10-15 minutes before carving.
11. With a sharp knife, cut the chicken into desired sized pieces and serve.
12. Serving Suggestions: Roasted vegetables will accompany this roasted chicken nicely.
13. Variation Tip: Rub the chicken with your hands for even coating.

Nutrition Info: Calories: 434 Fat: 15g Sat Fat: 6.9g Carbohydrates: 2.5g Fiber: 0.9g Sugar: 0.5g Protein: 66.4g

Marinated Chicken Thighs

Servings: 4
Cooking Time: 30 Minutes

Ingredients:
- 4 (6-ounce) bone-in, skin-on chicken thighs
- Salt and freshly ground black pepper, to taste
- ½ cup Italian salad dressing
- 1 teaspoon onion powder
- 1 teaspoon garlic powder

Directions:
1. Season the chicken thighs with salt and black pepper evenly.
2. In a large bowl, add the chicken thighs and dressing and mix well.
3. Cover the bowl and refrigerate to marinate overnight.
4. Remove the chicken breast from the bowl and place onto a plate.
5. Sprinkle the chicken thighs with onion powder and garlic powder.
6. Press "Power Button" of Ninja Foodi Digital Air Fry Oven and turn the dial to select "Air Fry" mode.
7. Press "Time Button" and again turn the dial to set the cooking time to 30 minutes.
8. Now push "Temp Button" and rotate the dial to set the temperature at 360 degrees F.
9. Press "Start/Pause" button to start.
10. When the unit beeps to show that it is preheated, open the lid and grease the air fry basket.
11. Arrange the chicken thighs into the prepared basket and insert in the oven.
12. After 15 minutes of cooking, flip the chicken thighs once.
13. When cooking time is complete, open the lid and transfer the chicken thighs onto serving plates.
14. Serve hot.
15. Serving Suggestions: Enjoy with honey glazed baby carrots.
16. Variation Tip: Select the chicken thighs with a pinkish hue.

Nutrition Info: Calories: 413 Fat: 21g Sat Fat: 4.8g Carbohydrates: 4.1g Fiber: 0.1g Sugar: 2.8g Protein: 49.5g

Glazed Turkey Breast

Servings: 10
Cooking Time: 55 Minutes

Ingredients:
- 1 teaspoon dried thyme, crushed
- ½ teaspoon dried sage, crushed
- ½ teaspoon smoked paprika
- Salt and freshly ground black pepper, to taste
- 1 (5-pound) boneless turkey breast
- 2 teaspoons olive oil
- ¼ cup maple syrup
- 2 tablespoons Dijon mustard
- 1 tablespoon butter, softened

Directions:
1. In a bowl, mix together the herbs, paprika, salt, and black pepper.
2. Coat the turkey breast with oil evenly.
3. Now, coat the outer side of turkey breast with herb mixture.
4. Press "Power Button" of Ninja Foodi Digital Air Fry Oven and turn the dial to select "Air Fry" mode.
5. Press "Time Button" and again turn the dial to set the cooking time to 55 minutes.
6. Now push "Temp Button" and rotate the dial to set the temperature at 350 degrees F.
7. Press "Start/Pause" button to start.
8. When the unit beeps to show that it is preheated, open the lid and grease the air fry basket.
9. Arrange the turkey breast into the prepared basket and insert in the oven.
10. While cooking, flip the turkey breast once after 25 minutes and then after 37 minutes.
11. Meanwhile, in a bowl, mix together the maple syrup, mustard, and butter.
12. After 50 minutes of cooking, press "Start/Pause" to pause cooking.
13. Remove the basket from Air Fryer and coat the turkey breast with glaze evenly.
14. Again, insert the basket in the oven and press "Start/Pause" to resume cooking.
15. When cooking time is complete, open the lid and place the turkey breast onto a cutting board for about 10 minutes before slicing.
16. With a sharp knife, cut the turkey breast into desired sized slices and serve.
17. Serving Suggestions: Green bean and goats cheese salad will be best for turkey meat.
18. Variation Tip: Place the turkey into the basket with the breast side down.

Nutrition Info: Calories: 30w, Fat: 3.3g, Sat Fat: 0.9g, Carbohydrates: 5.6g, Fiber: 0.2g Sugar: 4.7g, Protein: 26.2g

MEAT RECIPES
Bbq Baby Ribs

Servings: 4
Cooking Time: 35 Minutes

Ingredients:
- 3 lb. ribs of baby back pork
- 1 tablespoon each of white and brown sugar
- 1 teaspoon smoked paprika
- 1 teaspoon of garlic, granulated
- 1/3 cup barbeque sauce

Directions:
1. Preheat your air fryer to 175 degrees C or 350 degrees F.
2. Strip off the membrane from the rib's back. Cut into 4 equal size portions.
3. Bring together the brown and white sugar, paprika, pepper, granulated garlic, and the green seasoning (optional) in a bowl.
4. Rub the spice mix all over your pork ribs.
5. Keep in the fryer basket.
6. Now cook the ribs for 25 minutes. Turn once after 12 minutes.
7. Brush the BBQ sauce.
8. Air fry this for another 5 minutes.

Nutrition Info: Calories 752, Carbohydrates 16g, Cholesterol 176mg, Total Fat 60g, Fiber 0.7g, Protein 37g, Sugar 12g, Sodium 415mg

Buttered Leg Of Lamb

Servings: 8
Cooking Time: 1¼ Hours

Ingredients:
- 1 (2¼-pound) boneless leg of lamb
- 3 tablespoons butter, melted
- Salt and freshly ground black pepper, to taste
- 4 fresh rosemary sprigs

Directions:
1. Rub the leg of lamb with butter and sprinkle with salt and black pepper.
2. Wrap the leg of lamb with rosemary sprigs.
3. Press "Power Button" of Ninja Foodi Digital Air Fry Oven and turn the dial to select "Air Fry" mode.
4. Press "Time Button" and again turn the dial to set the cooking time to 75 minutes.
5. Now push "Temp Button" and rotate the dial to set the temperature at 300 degrees F.
6. Press "Start/Pause" button to start.
7. When the unit beeps to show that it is preheated, open the lid and grease air fry basket.
8. Arrange the leg of lamb into the air fry basket and insert in the oven.
9. When cooking time is complete, open the lid and place the leg of lamb onto a cutting board for about 10 minutes before slicing.
10. Cut into desired sized pieces and serve.
11. Serving Suggestions: Dijon mustard glazed carrots will be great if served with le
12. Variation Tip: You can add spices of your choice for seasoning of the leg of lamb.

Nutrition Info: Calories: 278 Fat: 13.8g Sat Fat: 6.1g Carbohydrates: 0.5g Fiber: 0.4g Sugar: 0g Protein: 35.9g

Mushrooms With Steak

Servings: 4
Cooking Time: 10 Minutes

Ingredients:
- 1 oz. sirloin beef steak, cut into small 1-inch cubes
- ¼ cup Worcestershire sauce
- 8 oz. sliced button mushrooms
- 1 tablespoon of olive oil
- 1 teaspoon chili flakes, crushed

Directions:
1. Combine the mushrooms, steak, olive oil Worcestershire sauce, and chili flakes in your bowl.
2. Keep it refrigerated for 4 hours minimum.
3. Take out 30 minutes before cooking.
4. Preheat your oven to 200 degrees C or 400 degrees F.
5. Drain out the marinade from your steak mixture.
6. Now keep the mushrooms and steak in the air fryer basket.
7. Cook for 5 minutes in the air fryer.
8. Toss and then cook for another 5 minutes.
9. Transfer the mushrooms and steak to a serving plate.

Nutrition Info: Calories 261, Carbohydrates 6g, Cholesterol 60mg, Total Fat 17g, Protein 21g, Sugar 3g, Fiber 0.9g, Sodium 213mg

Braised Lamb Shanks

Servings: 4
Cooking Time: 2 Hours, 30 Minutes
Ingredients:
- 4 lamb shanks
- 4 crushed garlic cloves
- 2 tablespoons of olive oil
- 3 cups of beef broth
- 2 tablespoons balsamic vinegar

Directions:
1. Rub pepper and salt on your lamb shanks. Keep in the baking pan.
2. Rub the smashed garlic on the lamb well.
3. Now cut the shanks with olive oil.
4. Keep underneath your lamb.
5. Keep the pan into the rack.
6. Roast for 20 minutes at 425 degrees F. Change to low for 2 hours at 250 F.
7. Add vinegar and 2 cups of broth.
8. Including the remaining broth after the 1st hour.

Nutrition Info: Calories 453, Carbohydrates 6g, Cholesterol 121mg, Total Fat 37g, Protein 24g, Fiber 2g, Sodium 578mg

Glazed Lamb Meatballs

Servings: 8
Cooking Time: 30 Minutes

Ingredients:
- For Meatballs:
- 2 pounds lean ground lamb
- 2/3 cup quick-cooking oats
- ½ cup Ritz crackers, crushed
- 1 (5-ounce) can evaporated milk
- 2 large eggs, beaten lightly
- 1 teaspoon maple syrup
- 1 tablespoon dried onion, minced
- Salt and freshly ground black pepper, to taste
- For Sauce:
- 1/3 cup orange marmalade
- 1/3 cup maple syrup
- 1/3 cup sugar
- 2 tablespoons cornstarch
- 2 tablespoons soy sauce
- 1-2 tablespoons Sriracha
- 1 tablespoon Worcestershire sauce

Directions:
1. For meatballs: in a large bowl, add all the ingredients and mix until well combined.
2. Make 1½-inch balls from the mixture.
3. Arrange half of the meatballs onto the greased sheet pan in a single layer.
4. Press "Power Button" of Ninja Foodi Digital Air Fry Oven and turn the dial to select "Air Fry" mode.
5. Press "Time Button" and again turn the dial to set the cooking time to 15 minutes.
6. Now push "Temp Button" and rotate the dial to set the temperature at 380 degrees F.
7. Press "Start/Pause" button to start.
8. When the unit beeps to show that it is preheated, open the lid and insert the sheet pan in the oven.
9. Flip the meatballs once halfway through.
10. When cooking time is complete, open the lid and transfer the meatballs into a bowl.
11. Repeat with the remaining meatballs.
12. Meanwhile, for sauce: in a small pan, add all the ingredients over medium heat and cook until thickened, stirring continuously.
13. Serve the meatballs with the topping of sauce.
14. Serving Suggestions: Mashed buttery potatoes make a classic pairing with meatballs.
15. Variation Tip: You can adjust the ratio of sweetener according to your taste.

Nutrition Info: Calories: 413, Fat: 11.9g, Sat Fat: 4.3g Carbohydrates: 39.5g, Fiber: 1g Sugar: 28.2g, Protein: 36.2g

Sweet Potato, Brown Rice, And Lamb

Servings: 2
Cooking Time: 10 Minutes

Ingredients:
- ¼ cup lamb, cooked and puréed
- ½ cup cooked brown rice
- ¼ cup of sweet potato purée

Directions:
1. Keep all the ingredients in your bowl.
2. Pulse until you achieve the desired consistency.
3. Process with milk to get a smoother consistency.
4. Store in an airtight container. Refrigerate.

Nutrition Info: Calories 37, Carbohydrates 5g, Cholesterol 7mg, Total Fat 1g, Protein 2g, Fiber 1g, Sodium 6mg

Buttered Rib Eye Steak

Servings: 3
Cooking Time: 14 Minutes

Ingredients:
- 2 (8-ounce) rib eye steaks
- 2 tablespoons butter, melted
- Salt and ground black pepper, as required

Directions:
1. Coat the steak with butter and then, sprinkle with salt and black pepper evenly.
2. Press "Power Button" of Ninja Foodi Digital Air Fry Oven and turn the dial to select the "Air Roast" mode.
3. Press the Time button and again turn the dial to set the cooking time to 14 minutes.
4. Now push the Temp button and rotate the dial to set the temperature at 400 degrees F.
5. Press "Start/Pause" button to start.
6. When the unit beeps to show that it is preheated, open the lid and grease "Air Fry Basket".
7. Arrange the steaks into "Air Fry Basket" and insert in the oven.
8. Remove from the oven and place steaks onto a platter for about 5 minutes.
9. Cut each steak into desired size slices and serve.

Nutrition Info: Calories 388 Total Fat 23.7 g Saturated Fat 110.2 g Cholesterol 154 mg Sodium 278 mg Total Carbs 0 g Fiber 0 g Sugar 0 g Protein 41 g

Beef Kabobs

Servings: 4
Cooking Time: 10 Minutes

Ingredients:
- 1 oz. beef ribs, cut into small 1-inch pieces
- 2 tablespoons soy sauce
- 1/3 cup low-fat sour cream
- 1 bell pepper
- ½ onion

Directions:
1. Mix soy sauce and sour cream in a bowl.
2. Keep the chunks of beef in the bowl. Marinate for 30 minutes' minimum.
3. Now cut the onion and bell pepper into one-inch pieces.
4. Soak 8 skewers in water.
5. Thread the bell pepper, onions, and beef on the skewers. Add some pepper.
6. Cook for 10 minutes in your pre-heated air fryer. Turn after 5 minutes.

Nutrition Info: Calories 297, Carbohydrates 4g, Cholesterol 84mg, Total Fat 21g, Protein 23g, Sugar 2g, Sodium 609mg, Calcium 49mg

Bacon-wrapped Filet Mignon

Servings: 2
Cooking Time: 15 Minutes

Ingredients:
- 2 bacon slices
- 2 (4-ounce) filet mignon
- Salt and freshly ground black pepper, to taste
- Olive oil cooking spray

Directions:
1. Wrap 1 bacon slice around each filet mignon and secure with toothpicks.
2. Season the filets with the salt and black pepper lightly.
3. Press "Power Button" of Ninja Foodi Digital Air Fry Oven and turn the dial to select "Air Fry" mode.
4. Press "Time Button" and again turn the dial to set the cooking time to 15 minutes.
5. Now push "Temp Button" and rotate the dial to set the temperature at 375 degrees F.
6. Press "Start/Pause" button to start.
7. When the unit beeps to show that it is preheated, open the lid.
8. Arrange the filets over the greased rack and insert in the oven.
9. Flip the filets once halfway through.
10. When cooking time is complete, open the lid and transfer the filets onto serving plates.
11. Serve hot.
12. Serving Suggestions: Fresh baby greens will accompany these filets greatly.
13. Variation Tip: Don't forget to secure the wrapped meat with toothpicks.

Nutrition Info: Calories: 226 Fat: 9.5g Sat Fat: g3.6 Carbohydrates: 0g Fiber: 0g Sugar: 0g Protein: 33.3g

Stuffed Pork Roll

Servings: 4
Cooking Time: 20 Minutes

Ingredients:
- 1 scallion, chopped
- ¼ cup sun-dried tomatoes, chopped finely
- 2 tablespoons fresh parsley, chopped
- Salt and freshly ground black pepper, to taste
- 4 (6-ounce) pork cutlets, pounded slightly
- 2 teaspoons paprika
- ½ tablespoons olive oil

Directions:
1. In a bowl, mix together the scallion, tomatoes, parsley, salt, and black pepper.
2. Spread the tomato mixture over each pork cutlet.
3. Roll each cutlet and secure with cocktail sticks.
4. Rub the outer part of rolls with paprika, salt and black pepper.
5. Coat the rolls with oil evenly.
6. Press "Power Button" of Ninja Foodi Digital Air Fry Oven and turn the dial to select "Air Fry" mode.
7. Press "Time Button" and again turn the dial to set the cooking time to 15 minutes.
8. Now push "Temp Button" and rotate the dial to set the temperature at 390 degrees F.
9. Press "Start/Pause" button to start.
10. When the unit beeps to show that it is preheated, open the lid and grease air fry basket.
11. Arrange pork rolls into the prepared air fry basket in a single layer and insert in the oven.
12. When cooking time is complete, open the lid and transfer the pork rolls onto serving plates.
13. Serve hot.
14. Serving Suggestions: Serve these pork rolls with creamed spinach.
15. Variation Tip: Drain the sun-dried tomatoes completely before using them.

Nutrition Info: Calories: 244 Fat: 14.5g Sat Fat: 2.7g Carbohydrates: 20.1g Fiber: 2.6g Sugar: 1.7g Protein: 8.2g

Almonds Crusted Rack Of Lamb

Servings: 5
Cooking Time: 35 Minutes

Ingredients:
- 1 tablespoon olive oil
- 1 garlic clove, minced
- Salt and freshly ground black pepper, to taste
- 1 (1¾-pound) rack of lamb
- 1 egg
- 1 tablespoon breadcrumbs
- 3 ounces almonds, finely chopped

Directions:
1. In a bowl, mix together the oil, garlic, salt, and black pepper.
2. Coat the rack of lamb evenly with oil mixture.
3. Crack the egg in a shallow bowl and beat well.
4. In another bowl, mix together the breadcrumbs and almonds.
5. Dip the rack of lamb in beaten egg and then, coat with almond mixture.
6. Press "Power Button" of Ninja Foodi Digital Air Fry Oven and turn the dial to select "Air Fry" mode.
7. Press "Time Button" and again turn the dial to set the cooking time to 30 minutes.
8. Now push "Temp Button" and rotate the dial to set the temperature at 220 degrees F.
9. Press "Start/Pause" button to start.
10. When the unit beeps to show that it is preheated, open the lid and grease air fry basket.
11. Place the rack of lamb into the prepared air fry basket and insert in the oven.
12. After 30 minutes, set the temperature of to 390 degrees F for 5 minutes.
13. When cooking time is complete, open the lid and place the rack of lamb onto a cutting board for about 5 minutes.
14. With a sharp knife, cut the rack of lamb into individual chops and serve.
15. Serving Suggestions: Serve with a fresh spinach salad.
16. Variation Tip: For best result, remove the silver skin from rack of lamb.

Nutrition Info: Calories: 408 Fat: 26.3g Sat Fat: 6.3g Carbohydrates: 4.9g Fiber: 2.2g Sugar: 0.9g Protein: 37.2g

Ranch Pork Chops

Servings: 4
Cooking Time: 15 Minutes

Ingredients:
- 4 pork chops, boneless and center-cut
- 2 teaspoons salad dressing mix

Directions:
1. Keep your pork chops on a plate.
2. Apply cooking spray on both sides lightly.
3. Sprinkle the seasoning mixture on both sides.
4. Allow to sit at room temperature for 5 minutes.
5. Apply cooking spray on the basket.
6. Preheat your air fryer to 200 degrees C or 390 degrees F.
7. Keep the chops in the air fryer. It shouldn't get overcrowded.
8. Cook for 5 minutes. Now flip your chops and cook for another 5 minutes.
9. Allow it to rest before serving.

Nutrition Info: Calories 276, Carbohydrates 1g, Cholesterol 107mg, Total Fat 12g, Fiber 0g, Protein 41g, Sugar 0g, Sodium 148mg

Beef Chuck Roast

Servings: 6
Cooking Time: 45 Minutes

Ingredients:
- 1 (2-pound) beef chuck roast
- 1 tablespoon olive oil
- 1 teaspoon dried rosemary, crushed
- 1 teaspoon dried thyme, crushed
- Salt, as required

Directions:
1. In a bowl, add the oil, herbs and salt and mix well.
2. Coat the beef roast with herb mixture generously.
3. Arrange the beef roast onto the greased cooking pan.
4. Press "Power Button" of Ninja Foodi Digital Air Fry Oven and turn the dial to select the "Air Fry" mode.
5. Press the Time button and again turn the dial to set the cooking time to 45 minutes.
6. Now push the Temp button and rotate the dial to set the temperature at 360 degrees F.
7. Press "Start/Pause" button to start.
8. When the unit beeps to show that it is preheated, open the lid and insert baking pan in the oven.
9. Remove from oven and place the roast onto a cutting board.
10. With a piece of foil, cover the beef roast for about 20 minutes before slicing.
11. With a sharp knife, cut the beef roast into desired size slices and serve.

Nutrition Info: Calories 304 Total Fat 14 g Saturated Fat 4.5 g Cholesterol 130 mg Sodium 82 mg Total Carbs 0.2g Fiber 0.2 g Sugar 0 g Protein 41.5 g

Lamb Sirloin Steak

Servings: 4
Cooking Time: 15 Minutes

Ingredients:
- 1 oz. lamb sirloin steaks, boneless
- 5 garlic cloves
- 1 teaspoon fennel, ground
- ½ onion
- 1 teaspoon cinnamon, ground

Directions:
1. Add all the ingredients in your blender bowl other than the lamb chops.
2. Pulse and blend until you see the onion minced fine. All the ingredients should be blended well.
3. Now keep your lamb chops in a big-sized bowl.
4. Slash the meat and fat with a knife.
5. The marinade should penetrate.
6. Include the spice paste. Mix well.
7. Refrigerate the mixture for half an hour.
8. Keep the steaks of lamb in your air fryer basket.
9. Cook, flipping once.

Nutrition Info: Calories 189, Carbohydrates 3g, Total Fat 9g, Protein 24g, Fiber 1g

Spiced Flank Steak

Servings: 6
Cooking Time: 12 Minutes

Ingredients:
- 2 tablespoons balsamic vinegar
- 2 tablespoons olive oil
- 3 garlic cloves, minced
- 1 teaspoon red chili powder
- 1 teaspoon ground cumin
- 1 teaspoon onion powder
- Salt and freshly ground black pepper, to taste
- 1 (2-pound) flank steak

Directions:
1. In a large bowl, mix together the vinegar, spices, salt and black pepper.
2. Add the steak and coat with mixture generously.
3. Cover the bowl and place in the refrigerator for at least 1 hour.
4. Remove the steak from bowl and place onto the greased sheet pan.
5. Press "Power Button" of Ninja Foodi Digital Air Fry Oven and turn the dial to select the "Air Broil" mode.
6. Press "Time Button" and again turn the dial to set the cooking time to 12 minutes.
7. Press "Start/Pause" button to start.
8. When the unit beeps to show that it is preheated, open the lid and insert the sheet pan in the oven.
9. Flip the steak once halfway through.
10. When cooking time is complete, open the lid and place the steak onto a cutting board.
11. With a sharp knife, cut the steak into desired sized slices and serve.
12. Serving Suggestions: Enjoy this steak with a drizzling of fresh lemon juice.
13. Variation Tip: choose the steak that is as uniform in thickness.

Nutrition Info: Calories: 341 Fat: 17.4g Sat Fat: 5.9g Carbohydrates: 1.3g Fiber: 0.2g Sugar: 0.2g Protein: 42.3g

Italian-style Meatballs

Servings: 12
Cooking Time: 35 Minutes

Ingredients:
- 10 oz. lean beef, ground
- 3 garlic cloves, minced
- 5 oz. turkey sausage
- 2 tablespoons shallot, minced
- 1 large egg, lightly beaten
- 2 tablespoons of olive oil
- 1 tablespoon of rosemary and thyme, chopped

Directions:
1. Preheat your air fryer to 400 degrees F.
2. Heat oil and add the shallot. Cook for 1-2 minutes.
3. Add the garlic now and cook. Take out from the heat.
4. Add the garlic and cooked shallot along with the egg, turkey sausage, beef, rosemary, thyme, and salt. Combine well by stirring.
5. Shape the mixture gently into 1-1/2 inch small balls.
6. Keep the balls in your air fryer basket.
7. Cook your meatballs at 400 degrees F. They should turn light brown.
8. Take out. Keep warm.
9. Serve the meatballs over rice or pasta.

Nutrition Info: Calories 175, Carbohydrates 0g, Total Fat 15g, Fiber 0g, Protein 10g, Sugar 0g, Sodium 254mg

Glazed Lamb Chops

Servings: 4
Cooking Time: 15 Minutes

Ingredients:
- 1 tablespoon Dijon mustard
- ½ tablespoon fresh lime juice
- 1 teaspoon honey
- ½ teaspoon olive oil
- Salt and freshly ground black pepper, to taste
- 4 (4-ounce) lamb loin chops

Directions:
1. In a black pepper large bowl, mix together the mustard, lemon juice, oil, honey, salt, and black pepper.
2. Add the chops and coat with the mixture generously.
3. Place the chops onto the greased sheet pan.
4. Press "Power Button" of Ninja Foodi Digital Air Fry Oven and turn the dial to select "Air Bake" mode.
5. Press "Time Button" and again turn the dial to set the cooking time to 15 minutes.
6. Now push "Temp Button" and rotate the dial to set the temperature at 390 degrees F.
7. Press "Start/Pause" button to start.
8. When the unit beeps to show that it is preheated, open the lid and insert the sheet pan in the oven.
9. Flip the chops once halfway through.
10. When cooking time is complete, open the lid and transfer the chops onto serving plates.
11. Serve hot.
12. Serving Suggestions: Serve the chops with mashed potatoes or polenta.
13. Variation Tip: Remember to pat dry the chops before seasoning.

Nutrition Info: Calories: 224 Fat: 9.1g Sat Fat: 3.1g Carbohydrates: 1.7g Fiber: 0.1g Sugar: 1.5g Protein: 32g

Air-fried Meatloaf

Servings: 4
Cooking Time: 45 Minutes

Ingredients:
- 8 oz. pork, ground
- 8 oz. veal, ground
- 1 large egg
- ¼ cup bread crumbs
- 1.4 cup cilantro, chopped
- 1 teaspoon of olive oil
- 2 teaspoons chipotle chili sauce

Directions:
1. Preheat your air fryer to 200 degrees C or 400 degrees F.
2. Bring together the veal and pork in a baking dish. Make sure that it goes into your air fryer basket.
3. Create a well. Now add the cilantro, egg, bread crumbs, salt, and pepper.
4. Use your hands to mix well and create a loaf.
5. Combine the olive oil and chipotle chili sauce in a bowl. Whisk well.
6. Keep it aside.
7. Cook the meatloaf in your air fryer. Take it out and add the juicy mix.
8. Bring back the meatloaf to the fryer. Bake for 7 minutes.
9. Turn the fryer off. Allow the meatloaf to rest for 6 minutes inside.
10. Take it out and let it rest for 5 more minutes.
11. Slice before serving.

Nutrition Info: Calories 311, Carbohydrates 13g, Cholesterol 123mg, Total Fat 19g, Fiber 0.7g, Protein 22g, Sugar 8g, Sodium 536mg

VEGETARIAN AND VEGAN RECIPES
Broccoli With Cauliflower

Servings: 6
Cooking Time: 15 Minutes

Ingredients:
- 1-pound broccoli, cut into 1-inch florets
- 1-pound cauliflower, cut into 1-inch florets
- 2 tablespoons butter
- Salt and ground black pepper, as required
- ¼ cup Parmesan cheese, grated

Directions:
1. In a pan of the boiling water, add the broccoli and cook for about 3-4 minutes.
2. Drain the broccoli well.
3. In a bowl, place the broccoli, cauliflower, oil, salt, and black pepper and toss to coat well.
4. Press "Power Button" of Ninja Foodi Digital Air Fry Oven and turn the dial to select the "Air Fry" mode.
5. Press the Time button and again turn the dial to set the cooking time to 15 minutes.
6. Now push the Temp button and rotate the dial to set the temperature at 400 degrees F.
7. Press "Start/Pause" button to start.
8. When the unit beeps to show that it is preheated, open the lid.
9. Arrange the veggie mixture in "Air Fry Basket" and insert in the oven.
10. Toss the veggie mixture once halfway through.
11. Remove from oven and transfer the veggie mixture into a large bowl.
12. Immediately, stir in the cheese and serve immediately.

Nutrition Info: Calories 91 Total Fat 5 g Saturated Fat 2.8 g Cholesterol 13 mg Sodium 131 mg Total Carbs 9 g Fiber 3.9 g Sugar 3.1 g Protein 5 g

Air Fryer Pumpkin Keto Pancakes

Servings: 2
Cooking Time: 5 Minutes

Ingredients:
- ½ cup pumpkin puree
- 1 teaspoon of vanilla extract
- 2 eggs
- ½ cup peanut butter
- ½ teaspoon baking soda

Directions:
1. Use parchment paper to line the basket of your air fryer.
2. Apply some cooking spray.
3. Bring together the eggs, peanut butter, pumpkin puree, baking soda, salt, and eggs in a bowl. Combine well by stirring.
4. Place 3 tablespoons of the batter in each pancake. There should be a half-inch space between them.
5. Keep the basket in your air fryer oven.
6. Cook for 4 minutes at 150 degrees C or 300 degrees F.

Nutrition Info: Calories 586, Carbohydrates 20g, Cholesterol 186mg, Total Fat 46g, Protein 23g, Sugar 9g, Fiber 6g, Sodium 906mg

Basil Tomatoes

Servings: 2
Cooking Time: 10 Minutes

Ingredients:
- 3 tomatoes, halved
- Olive oil cooking spray
- Salt and freshly ground black pepper, to taste
- 1 tablespoon fresh basil, chopped

Directions:
1. Drizzle the cut sides of the tomato halves with cooking spray evenly.
2. Then, sprinkle with salt, black pepper and basil.
3. Press "Power Button" of Ninja Foodi Digital Air Fry Oven and turn the dial to select "Air Fry" mode.
4. Press "Time Button" and again turn the dial to set the cooking time to 10 minutes.
5. Now push "Temp Button" and rotate the dial to set the temperature at 320 degrees F.
6. Press "Start/Pause" button to start.
7. When the unit beeps to show that it is preheated, open the lid.
8. Arrange the tomatoes into the air fry basket and insert in the oven.
9. When cooking time is complete, open the lid and transfer the tomatoes onto serving plates.
10. Serve warm.
11. Serving Suggestions: You can use these tomatoes in pasta and pasta salads with a drizzle of balsamic vinegar.
12. Variation Tip: Fresh thyme can also be used instead of basil.

Nutrition Info: Calories: 34 Fat: 0.4g Sat Fat: 0.1g Carbohydrates: 7.2g Fiber: 2.2g Sugar: 4.9g Protein: 1.7g

Buttered Veggies

Servings: 3
Cooking Time: 20 Minutes

Ingredients:
- 1 cup potatoes, chopped
- 1 cup beets, peeled and chopped
- 1 cup carrots, peeled and chopped
- 2 garlic cloves, minced
- Salt and ground black pepper, as required
- 3 tablespoons olive oil

Directions:
1. In a bowl, place all ingredients and toss to coat well.
2. Place the tofu mixture in the greased "Sheet Pan".
3. Press "Power Button" of Ninja Foodi Digital Air Fry Oven and turn the dial to select the "Air Bake" mode.
4. Press the Time button and again turn the dial to set the cooking time to 20 minutes.
5. Now push the Temp button and rotate the dial to set the temperature at 450 degrees F.
6. Press "Start/Pause" button to start.
7. When the unit beeps to show that it is preheated, open the lid.
8. Insert the "Sheet Pan" in oven.
9. Toss the veggie mixture once halfway through.
10. Serve hot.

Nutrition Info: Calories 197 Total Fat 14.2 g Saturated Fat 2 g Cholesterol 0 mg Sodium 123 mg Total Carbs 17.8 g Fiber 3.3 g Sugar 6.9 g Protein 2.2 g

Potato Tots

Servings: 24
Cooking Time: 35 Minutes

Ingredients:
- 2 peeled sweet potatoes
- Olive oil cooking spray
- ½ teaspoon Cajun seasoning
- Sea salt to taste

Directions:
1. Boil a pot of water. Add the sweet potatoes in it.
2. Keep boiling until you can pierce them using a fork.
3. It should take about 15 minutes. Don't over boil, as they can get too messy for grating. Drain off the liquid. Allow it to cool.
4. Grate the potatoes in a bowl.
5. Now mix your Cajun seasoning carefully.
6. Create tot-shaped cylinders with this mixture.
7. Spray some olive oil on your fryer basket.
8. Keep the tots in it. They should be in 1 row and shouldn't be touching each other or the basket's sides.
9. Apply some olive oil spray on the tots.
10. Heat your air fryer to 200 degrees C or 400 degrees F.
11. Cook for 8 minutes.
12. Flip over and cook for 8 more minutes after applying the olive oil spray again.

Nutrition Info: Calories 22, Carbohydrates 5g, Cholesterol 0mg, Total Fat 0g, Protein 0.4g, Sugar 1g, Fiber 0.7g, Sodium 36mg

Corn Nuts

Servings: 8
Cooking Time: 25 Minutes

Ingredients:
- 1 oz. white corn
- 1-1/2 teaspoons salt
- 3 tablespoons of vegetable oil

Directions:
1. Keep the corn in a bowl. Cover this with water. Keep aside for 8 hours minimum for hydration.
2. Drain the corn. Spread it on a baking sheet. They should be in an even layer.
3. Use paper towels to pat dry. Also air dry for 15 minutes.
4. Preheat your air fryer to 200 degrees C or 400 degrees F.
5. Transfer the corn to a bowl. Add salt and oil. Stir to coat evenly.
6. Keep the corn in your air fryer basket in an even layer.
7. Cook for 8 minutes.
8. Shake the basket and cook for 8 minutes more.
9. Shake the basket once more. Cook for 5 more minutes.
10. Transfer to a plate lined with a paper towel.
11. Set aside for allowing the corn nuts to cool. They should be crisp.

Nutrition Info: Calories 240, Carbohydrates 36g, Cholesterol 0mg, Total Fat 8g, Protein 6g, Sugar 1g, Fiber 7g, Sodium 438mg

Green Beans & Mushroom Casserole

Servings: 6
Cooking Time: 12 Minutes

Ingredients:
- 24 ounces fresh green beans, trimmed
- 2 cups fresh button mushrooms, sliced
- 3 tablespoons olive oil
- 2 tablespoons fresh lemon juice
- 1 teaspoon ground sage
- 1 teaspoon garlic powder
- 1 teaspoon onion powder
- Salt and freshly ground black pepper, to taste
- 1/3 cup French fried onions

Directions:
1. In a bowl, add the green beans, mushrooms, oil, lemon juice, sage, and spices and toss to coat well.
2. Press "Power Button" of Ninja Foodi Digital Air Fry Oven and turn the dial to select "Air Fry" mode.
3. Press "Time Button" and again turn the dial to set the cooking time to 12 minutes.
4. Now push "Temp Button" and rotate the dial to set the temperature at 400 degrees F.
5. Press "Start/Pause" button to start.
6. When the unit beeps to show that it is preheated, open the lid and grease the air fry basket.
7. Arrange the mushroom mixture into the prepared air fry basket and insert in the oven.
8. Shake the mushroom mixture occasionally.
9. When cooking time is complete, open the lid and transfer the mushroom mixture into a serving dish.
10. Top with fried onions and serve.
11. Serving Suggestions: Fresh salad will accompany this casserole nicely.
12. Variation Tip: Any kind of fresh mushrooms can be used.

Nutrition Info: Calories: 125 Fat: 8.6g Sat Fat: 2g Carbohydrates: 11g Fiber: 4.2g Sugar: 2.4g Protein: 3g

Veggie Kabobs

Servings: 6
Cooking Time: 10 Minutes

Ingredients:
- ¼ cup carrots, peeled and chopped
- ¼ cup French beans
- ½ cup green peas
- 1 teaspoon ginger
- 3 garlic cloves, peeled
- 3 green chilies
- ¼ cup fresh mint leaves
- ½ cup cottage cheese
- 2 medium boiled potatoes, mashed
- ½ teaspoon five-spice powder
- Salt, to taste
- 2 tablespoons corn flour
- Olive oil cooking spray

Directions:
1. In a food processor, add the carrot, beans, peas, ginger, garlic, mint, cheese and pulse until smooth.
2. Transfer the mixture into a bowl.
3. Add the mashed potatoes, five-spice powder, salt and corn flour and with your hands mix until well combined.
4. Shape the mixture into equal-sized small balls.
5. Press each ball around a skewer in a sausage shape.
6. Spray the skewers with cooking spray.
7. Press "Power Button" of Ninja Foodi Digital Air Fry Oven and turn the dial to select "Air Fry" mode.
8. Press "Time Button" and again turn the dial to set the cooking time to 10 minutes.
9. Now push "Temp Button" and rotate the dial to set the temperature at 390 degrees F.
10. Press "Start/Pause" button to start.
11. When the unit beeps to show that it is preheated, open the lid and grease the air fry basket.
12. Arrange the skewers into the prepared air fry basket and insert in the oven.
13. When cooking time is complete, open the lid and transfer the skewers onto a platter.
14. Serve warm.
15. Serving Suggestions: Enjoy these kabobs wt yogurt dip.
16. Variation Tip: You can add spices of your choice in these veggie kabobs

Nutrition Info: Calories: 120, Fat: 0.8g Sat Fat: 0.3g, Carbohydrates: 21.9g Fiber: 4.9g Sugar: 1.8g Protein: 6.3g

Sweet & Tangy Mushrooms

Servings: 4
Cooking Time: 15 Minutes

Ingredients:
- ¼ cup soy sauce
- ¼ cup honey
- ¼ cup balsamic vinegar
- 2 garlic cloves, chopped finely
- ½ teaspoon red pepper flakes, crushed
- 18 ounces cremini mushrooms, halved

Directions:
1. In a bowl, place the soy sauce, honey, vinegar, garlic and red pepper flakes and mix well. Set aside.
2. Place the mushroom into the greased baking pan in a single layer.
3. Press "Power Button" of Ninja Foodi Digital Air Fry Oven and turn the dial to select the "Air Bake" mode.
4. Press the Time button and again turn the dial to set the cooking time to 15 minutes.
5. Now push the Temp button and rotate the dial to set the temperature at 350 degrees F.
6. Press "Start/Pause" button to start.
7. When the unit beeps to show that it is preheated, open the lid.
8. Insert the baking pan in oven.
9. After 8 minutes of cooking, place the honey mixture in baking pan and toss to coat well.
10. Serve hot.

Nutrition Info: Calories 113 Total Fat 0.2 g Saturated Fat 0 g Cholesterol 0 mg Sodium 9.8 mg Total Carbs 24.7 g Fiber 1 g Sugar 20 g Protein 4.4 g

Spicy Potato

Servings: 4
Cooking Time: 25 Minutes

Ingredients:
- 2 cups water
- 6 russet potatoes, peeled and cubed
- ½ tablespoon extra-virgin olive oil
- ½ of onion, chopped
- 1 tablespoon fresh rosemary, chopped
- 1 garlic clove, minced
- 1 jalapeño pepper, chopped
- ½ teaspoon garam masala powder
- ¼ teaspoon ground cumin
- ¼ teaspoon red chili powder
- Salt and ground black pepper, as required

Directions:
1. In a large bowl, add the water and potatoes and set aside for about 30 minutes.
2. Drain well and pat dry with the paper towels.
3. In a bowl, add the potatoes and oil and toss to coat well.
4. Press "Power Button" of Ninja Foodi Digital Air Fry Oven and turn the dial to select the "Air Fry" mode.
5. Press the Time button and again turn the dial to set the cooking time to 5 minutes.
6. Now push the Temp button and rotate the dial to set the temperature at 330 degrees F.
7. Press "Start/Pause" button to start.
8. When the unit beeps to show that it is preheated, open the lid.
9. Arrange the potato cubes in "Air Fry Basket" and insert in the oven.
10. Remove from oven and transfer the potatoes into a bowl.
11. Add the remaining ingredients and toss to coat well.
12. Press "Power Button" of Ninja Foodi Digital Air Fry Oven and turn the dial to select the "Air Fry" mode.
13. Press the Time button and again turn the dial to set the cooking time to 20 minutes.
14. Now push the Temp button and rotate the dial to set the temperature at 390 degrees F.
15. Press "Start/Pause" button to start.
16. When the unit beeps to show that it is preheated, open the lid.
17. Arrange the potato mixture in "Air Fry Basket" and insert in the oven.
18. Serve hot.

Nutrition Info: Calories 274 Total Fat 2.3 g Saturated Fat 0.4 g Cholesterol 0 mg Sodium 65mg Total Carbs 52.6 g Fiber 8.5 g Sugar 4.4 g Protein 5.7 g

Glazed Mushrooms

Servings: 4
Cooking Time: 15 Minutes

Ingredients:
- ¼ cup soy sauce
- ¼ cup honey
- ¼ cup balsamic vinegar
- 2 garlic cloves, chopped finely
- ½ teaspoon red pepper flakes, crushed
- 18 ounces fresh Cremini mushrooms, halved

Directions:
1. In a bowl, place the soy sauce, honey, vinegar, garlic and red pepper flakes and mix well. Set aside.
2. Place the mushroom into the greased baking pan in a single layer.
3. Press "Power Button" of Ninja Foodi Digital Air Fry Oven and turn the dial to select "Air Bake" mode.
4. Press "Time Button" and again turn the dial to set the cooking time to 15 minutes.
5. Now push "Temp Button" and rotate the dial to set the temperature at 350 degrees F.
6. Press "Start/Pause" button to start.
7. When the unit beeps to show that it is preheated, open the lid.
8. Insert the baking pan in oven.
9. After 8 minutes of cooking, place the honey mixture in baking pan and toss to coat well.
10. When cooking time is complete, open the lid and transfer the mushrooms onto serving plates.
11. Serve hot.
12. Serving Suggestions: Topping of fresh chives or marjoram gives a delish touch to mushrooms.
13. Variation Tip: Maple syrup will be an excellent substitute for honey.

Nutrition Info: Calories: 113 Fat: 0.2g Sat Fat: 0g Carbohydrates: 24.7g Fiber: 1g Sugar: 20g Protein: 4.4g

Roasted Cauliflower And Broccoli

Servings: 6
Cooking Time: 15 Minutes

Ingredients:
- 3 cups cauliflower florets
- 3 cups of broccoli florets
- ¼ teaspoon of sea salt
- ½ teaspoon of garlic powder
- 2 tablespoons olive oil

Directions:
1. Preheat your air fryer to 200 degrees C or 400 degrees F.
2. Keep your florets of broccoli in a microwave-safe bowl.
3. Cook in your microwave for 3 minutes on high temperature. Drain off the accumulated liquid.
4. Now add the olive oil, cauliflower, sea salt, and garlic powder to the broccoli in the bowl.
5. Combine well by mixing.
6. Pour this mix now into your air fryer basket.
7. Cook for 10 minutes. Toss the vegetables after 5 minutes for even browning.

Nutrition Info: Calories 77, Carbohydrates 6g, Cholesterol 0mg, Total Fat 5g, Protein 2g, Sugar 2g, Fiber 3g, Sodium 103mg

Potato-skin Wedges

Servings: 4
Cooking Time: 30 Minutes

Ingredients:
- 4 medium potatoes
- 3 tablespoons of canola oil
- 1 cup of water
- ¼ teaspoon black pepper, ground
- 1 teaspoon paprika

Directions:
1. Keep the potatoes in a big-sized pot. Add salted water and keep covered. Boil.
2. Bring down the heat to medium. Let it simmer. It should become tender.
3. Drain the water on.
4. Keep in a bowl and place in the refrigerator until it becomes cool.
5. Bring together the paprika, oil, salt, and black pepper in a bowl.
6. Now cut the potatoes into small quarters. Toss them into your mixture.
7. Preheat your air fryer to 200 degrees C or 400 degrees F.
8. Add half of the wedges of potato into the fryer basket. Keep them skin-down. Don't overcrowd.
9. Cook for 15 minutes. It should become golden brown.

Nutrition Info: Calories 276, Carbohydrates 38g, Cholesterol 0mg, Total Fat 12g, Protein 4g, Sugar 2g, Fiber 5g, Sodium 160mg

Baked Potatoes

Servings: 2
Cooking Time: 1 Hour

Ingredients:
- 1 tablespoon peanut oil
- 2 large potatoes, scrubbed
- ½ teaspoon of coarse sea salt

Directions:
1. Preheat your air fryer to 200 degrees C or 400 degrees F.
2. Brush peanut oil on your potatoes.
3. Sprinkle some salt.
4. Keep them in the basket of your air fryer.
5. Cook the potatoes for an hour.

Nutrition Info: Calories 360, Carbohydrates 64g, Cholesterol 0mg, Total Fat 8g, Protein 8g, Sugar 3g, Fiber 8g, Sodium 462mg

Spicy Butternut Squash

Servings: 4
Cooking Time: 20 Minutes

Ingredients:
- 1 medium butternut squash, peeled, seeded and cut into chunk
- 2 teaspoons cumin seeds
- 1/8 teaspoon garlic powder
- 1/8 teaspoon chili flakes, crushed
- Salt and freshly ground black pepper, to taste
- 1 tablespoon olive oil
- 2 tablespoons pine nuts
- 2 tablespoons fresh cilantro, chopped

Directions:
1. In a bowl, mix together the squash, spices, and oil.
2. Press "Power Button" of Ninja Foodi Digital Air Fry Oven and turn the dial to select "Air Fry" mode.
3. Press "Time Button" and again turn the dial to set the cooking time to 20 minutes.
4. Now push "Temp Button" and rotate the dial to set the temperature at 375 degrees F.
5. Press "Start/Pause" button to start.
6. When the unit beeps to show that it is preheated, open the lid and grease the air fry basket.
7. Arrange the squash chunks into the prepared air fry basket and insert in the oven.
8. When cooking time is complete, open the lid and transfer the squash chunks onto serving plates.
9. Serve hot with the garnishing of pine nuts and cilantro.
10. Serving Suggestions: Serve with a sprinkle of sweet dried cranberries.
11. Variation Tip: you can microwave the butternut squash for 2-3 mins to make it softer and easier to remove the skin.

Nutrition Info: Calories: 191 Fat: 7g Sat Fat: 0.8g Carbohydrates: 34.3g Fiber: 6g Sugar: 6.4g Protein: 3.7g

Garlicky Brussels Sprout

Servings: 4
Cooking Time: 15 Minutes

Ingredients:
- 1 pound Brussels sprouts, cut in half
- 2 tablespoons oil
- 2 garlic cloves, minced
- ¼ teaspoon red pepper flakes, crushed
- Salt and freshly ground black pepper, to taste

Directions:
1. In a bowl, add all the ingredients and toss to coat well.
2. Press "Power Button" of Ninja Foodi Digital Air Fry Oven and turn the dial to select "Air Fry" mode.
3. Press "Time Button" and again turn the dial to set the cooking time to 12 minutes.
4. Now push "Temp Button" and rotate the dial to set the temperature at 390 degrees F.
5. Press "Start/Pause" button to start.
6. When the unit beeps to show that it is preheated, open the lid.
7. Arrange the Brussels sprouts into the air fry basket and insert in the oven.
8. When cooking time is complete, open the lid and transfer the Brussels sprouts onto serving plates.
9. Serve hot.
10. Serving Suggestions: Sprinkle with flaky sea salt before serving.
11. Variation Tip: Look for small to medium sprouts for better taste.

Nutrition Info: Calories: 113 Fat: 9g Sat Fat: 1.3g Carbohydrates: 8.3g Fiber: 2.6g Sugar: 4.2g Protein: 2.8g

Spicy Green Beans

Servings: 4
Cooking Time: 25 Minutes

Ingredients:
- ¾ oz. green beans, trimmed
- 1 teaspoon of soy sauce
- 1 tablespoon sesame oil
- 1 garlic clove, minced
- 1 teaspoon of rice wine vinegar

Directions:
1. Preheat your air fryer to 200 degrees C or 400 degrees F.
2. Keep the green beans in a bowl.
3. Whisk together the soy sauce, sesame oil, garlic, and rice wine vinegar in another bowl.
4. Pour the green beans into it.
5. Coat well by tossing. Leave it for 5 minutes to marinate.
6. Transfer half of the beans to your air fryer basket.
7. Cook for 12 minutes. Shake the basket after 6 minutes.
8. Repeat with the other portion of green beans.

Nutrition Info: Calories 81, Carbohydrates 7g, Cholesterol 0mg, Total Fat 5g, Protein 2g, Sugar 1g, Fiber 3g, Sodium 80mg

Stuffed Pumpkin

Servings: 2
Cooking Time: 30 Minutes

Ingredients:
- ½ pumpkin, small
- 1 sweet potato, diced
- 1 parsnip, diced
- 1 carrot, diced
- 1 egg

Directions:
1. Scrape out the seeds from the pumpkin.
2. Combine the sweet potato, parsnip, carrot, and the egg in a bowl.
3. Fill up your pumpkin with this vegetable mixture.
4. Preheat your air fryer to 175 degrees C or 350 degrees F.
5. Keep your stuffed pumpkin in the fryer's basket.
6. Cook for 25 minutes. It should become tender.

Nutrition Info: Calories 268, Carbohydrates 49g, Cholesterol 93mg, Total Fat 4g, Protein 9g, Sugar 13g, Fiber 10g, Sodium 210mg

SNACK & DESSERT RECIPES
Air-fried Butter Cake

Servings: 4
Cooking Time: 15 Minutes

Ingredients:
- 1 egg
- 7 tablespoons of butter, room temperature
- 1-2/3 cups all-purpose flour
- ½ cup white sugar
- 6 tablespoons of milk

Directions:
1. Preheat your air fryer to 180 degrees C or 350 degrees F.
2. Apply cooking spray on a small tube pan.
3. Beat ¼ cup and 2 tablespoons of butter. It should be creamy and light.
4. Include the egg. Mix until it gets fluffy and smooth.
5. Stir in the salt and flour now.
6. Add milk. Mix the batter thoroughly.
7. Transfer the batter to your pan. Level the surface with a spoon's back.
8. Keep this pan in the basket of your air fryer.
9. Bake until you see a toothpick coming out clean when inserted.
10. Take out the cake. Set aside for cooling for 5 minutes.

Nutrition Info: Calories 596, Carbohydrates 60g, Cholesterol 102mg, Total Fat 36g, Protein 8g, Sugar 20g, Fiber 1.4g, Sodium 210mg

Apple Fritters

Servings: 4
Cooking Time: 10 Minutes

Ingredients:
- 1 apple – cored, peeled, and chopped
- 1 cup all-purpose flour
- 1 egg
- ½ cup milk
- 1-1/2 teaspoons of baking powder
- 2 tablespoons white sugar

Directions:
1. Preheat your air fryer to 175 degrees C or 350 degrees F.
2. Keep parchment paper at the bottom of your fryer.
3. Apply cooking spray.
4. Mix together ¼ cup sugar, flour, baking powder, egg, milk, and salt in a bowl.
5. Combine well by stirring.
6. Sprinkle 2 tablespoons of sugar on the apples. Coat well.
7. Combine the apples into your flour mixture.
8. Use a cookie scoop and drop the fritters with it to the air fryer basket's bottom.
9. Now air fry for 5 minutes.
10. Flip the fritters once and fry for another 3 minutes. They should be golden.

Nutrition Info: Calories 307, Carbohydrates 65g, Cholesterol 48mg, Total Fat 3g, Protein 5g, Sugar 39g, Fiber 2g, Sodium 248mg

Crispy Coconut Prawns

Servings: 4
Cooking Time: 12 Minutes

Ingredients:
- ½ cup flour
- ¼ teaspoon paprika
- Salt and freshly ground white pepper, to taste
- 2 egg whites
- ¾ cup panko breadcrumbs
- ½ cup unsweetened coconut, shredded
- 2 teaspoons lemon zest, grated finely
- 1 pound prawns, peeled and deveined

Directions:
1. In a shallow dish, place the flour, paprika, salt and white pepper and mix well.
2. In a second shallow dish, add the egg whites and beat lightly.
3. In a third shallow dish, place the breadcrumbs, coconut and lemon zest and mix well.
4. Coat the prawns with flour mixture, then dip into egg whites and finally coat with the coconut mixture.
5. Place the prawns in the greased sheet pan.
6. Press "Power Button" of Ninja Foodi Digital Air Fry Oven and turn the dial to select "Air Bake" mode.
7. Press "Time Button" and again turn the dial to set the cooking time to 12 minutes.
8. Now push "Temp Button" and rotate the dial to set the temperature at 400 degrees F.
9. Press "Start/Pause" button to start.
10. When the unit beeps to show that it is preheated, open the lid and insert the sheet pan in the oven.
11. Flip the prawns once halfway through.
12. When cooking time is complete, open the lid and transfer the prawns onto a platter.
13. Serve hot.
14. Serving Suggestions: Sweet chili sauce will accompany these prawns nicely.
15. Variation Tip: You may use regular breadcrumbs instead of panko.

Nutrition Info: Calories: 310 Fat: 6.9g Sat Fat: 4.1g Carbohydrates: 18.7g Fiber: 1.5g Sugar: 0.9g Protein: 3.2g

Cheddar Biscuits

Servings: 8
Cooking Time: 10 Minutes

Ingredients:
- 1/3 cup unbleached all-purpose flour
- 1/8 teaspoon cayenne pepper
- 1/8 teaspoon smoked paprika
- Pinch of garlic powder
- Salt and freshly ground black pepper, to taste
- ½ cup sharp cheddar cheese, shredded
- 2 tablespoons butter, softened
- Nonstick cooking spray

Directions:
1. In a food processor, add the flour, spices, salt and black pepper and pulse until well combined.
2. Add the cheese and butter and pulse until a smooth dough forms.
3. Place the dough onto a lightly floured surface.
4. Make 16 small equal-sized balls from the dough and press each slightly.
5. Press "Power Button" of Ninja Foodi Digital Air Fry Oven and turn the dial to select "Air Bake" mode.
6. Press "Time Button" and again turn the dial to set the cooking time to 10 minutes.
7. Now push "Temp Button" and rotate the dial to set the temperature at 330 degrees F.
8. Press "Start/Pause" button to start.
9. When the unit beeps to show that it is preheated, open the lid and grease the air fry basket.
10. Arrange the biscuits into the prepared air fry basket and insert in the oven.
11. When cooking time is complete, open the lid and place the basket onto a wire rack for about 10 minutes.
12. Carefully invert the biscuits onto the wire rack to cool completely before serving.
13. Serving Suggestions: Serve these cheddar biscuits with the drizzling of garlic butter.
14. Variation Tip: For flaky layers, use cold butter.

Nutrition Info: Calories: 73 Fat: 5.3g Sat Fat: 3.3g Carbohydrates: 4.1g Fiber: 0.2g Sugar: 0.1g Protein: 2.3g

Vanilla Cheesecake

Servings: 6
Cooking Time: 14 Minutes

Ingredients:
- 1 cup honey graham cracker crumbs
- 2 tablespoons unsalted butter, softened
- 1 pound cream cheese, softened
- ½ cup sugar
- 2 large eggs

Directions:
1. Line a round baking pan with parchment paper.
2. For crust: in a bowl, add the graham cracker crumbs and butter.
3. Place the crust into the baking dish and press to smooth.
4. Press "Power Button" of Ninja Foodi Air Fry Oven and turn the dial to select the "Air Fry" mode.
5. Press "Time Button" and again turn the dial to set the cooking time to 4 minutes.
6. Now push "Temp Button" and rotate the dial to set the temperature at 350 degrees F.
7. Press "Start/Pause" button to start.
8. When the unit beeps to show that it is preheated, open the lid.
9. Arrange the baking pan of crust into the air fry basket and insert in the oven.
10. When cooking time is complete, open the lid and place the crust aside to cool for about 10 minutes.
11. Meanwhile, in a bowl, add the cream cheese and sugar and whisk until smooth.
12. Now, place the eggs, one at a time and whisk until the mixture becomes creamy.
13. Add the vanilla extract and mix well.
14. Place the cream cheese mixture over the crust evenly.
15. Press "Power Button" of Ninja Foodi Air Fry Oven and turn the dial to select the "Air Fry" mode.
16. Press "Time Button" and again turn the dial to set the cooking time to 10 minutes.
17. Now push "Temp Button" and rotate the dial to set the temperature at 350 degrees F.
18. Press "Start/Pause" button to start.
19. When the unit beeps to show that it is preheated, open the lid.
20. Arrange the baking pan into the air fry basket and insert in the oven.
21. When cooking time is complete, open the lid and place the pan onto a wire rack to cool completely.
22. Refrigerate overnight before serving.
23. Serving Suggestions: Serve with the topping of fresh berries.
24. Variation Tip: Your cream cheese should always be at room temperature.

Nutrition Info: Calories: 470 Fat: 33.9g, Sat Fat: 20.6g Carbohydrates: 349g, Fiber: 0.5g Sugar: 22g Protein: 9.4g

Fried Pickles

Servings: 8
Cooking Time: 10 Minutes

Ingredients:
- 2 tablespoons of sriracha sauce
- ½ cup mayonnaise
- 1 egg
- ½ cup all-purpose flour
- 2 tablespoons of milk
- ¼ teaspoon garlic powder
- 1 jar dill pickle chips

Directions:
1. Mix the sriracha sauce and mayonnaise together in a bowl.
2. Refrigerate until you can use it.
3. Heat your air fryer to 200 degrees C or 400 degrees F.
4. Drain the pickles. Use paper towels to dry them.
5. Now mix the milk and egg together in another bowl.
6. Also mix the cornmeal, flour, garlic powder, pepper, and salt in a third bowl.
7. Dip the pickle chips in your egg mix, and then in the flour mix. Coat both sides lightly. Press the mixture into chips lightly.
8. Apply cooking spray in the fryer basket.
9. Keep the chips in the fryer's basket.
10. Cook for 4 minutes. Flip over and cook for another 4 minutes.
11. Serve with the sriracha mayo.

Nutrition Info: Calories 198, Carbohydrates 15g, Cholesterol 26mg, Total Fat 14g, Protein 3g, Sugar 1g, Fiber 2g, Sodium 1024mg

Chocolate Mug Cake

Servings: 2
Cooking Time: 17 Minutes

Ingredients:

- ¼ cup flour
- 2 tablespoons sugar
- ¼ teaspoon baking powder
- 1/8 teaspoon baking soda
- 1/8 teaspoon salt
- 2 tablespoons milk
- 2 tablespoons applesauce
- ½ tablespoon vegetable oil
- ¼ teaspoon vanilla extract
- 2 tablespoons chocolate chips

Directions:

1. In a bowl, mix together the flour, sugar, baking powder, baking soda and salt.
2. Add the milk, applesauce, oil and vanilla extract and mix until well combined.
3. Gently, fold in the chocolate chips.
4. Place the mixture into an over proof mug.
5. Press "Power Button" of Ninja Foodi Digital Air Fry Oven and turn the dial to select "Air Bake" mode.
6. Press "Time Button" and again turn the dial to set the cooking time to 17 minutes.
7. Now push "Temp Button" and rotate the dial to set the temperature at 375 degrees F.
8. Press "Start/Pause" button to start.
9. When the unit beeps to show that it is preheated, open the lid.
10. Arrange the mug over the wire rack and insert in the oven.
11. When cooking time is complete, open the lid and place the mug onto a wire rack to cool for about 10 minutes.
12. Serve warm.
13. Serving Suggestions: Sprinkle the cake with powdered sugar before serving.
14. Variation Tip: Use the best quality chocolate chips for cake.

Nutrition Info: Calories: 204 Fat: 7g Sat Fat: 3.1g Carbohydrates: 33g Fiber: 1g Sugar: 19.8g Protein: 2.9g

Banana Split

Servings: 8
Cooking Time: 14 Minutes

Ingredients:
- 3 tablespoons coconut oil
- 1 cup panko breadcrumbs
- ½ cup corn flour
- 2 eggs
- 4 bananas, peeled and halved lengthwise
- 3 tablespoons sugar
- ¼ teaspoon ground cinnamon
- 2 tablespoons walnuts, chopped

Directions:
1. In a medium skillet, melt the coconut oil over medium heat and cook breadcrumbs for about 3-4 minutes or until golden browned and crumbled, stirring continuously.
2. Transfer the breadcrumbs into a shallow bowl and set aside to cool.
3. In a second bowl, place the corn flour.
4. In a third bowl, whisk the eggs.
5. Coat the banana slices with flour and then, dip into eggs and finally, coat with the breadcrumbs evenly.
6. In a small bowl, mix together the sugar and cinnamon.
7. Press "Power Button" of Ninja Foodi Digital Air Fry Oven and turn the dial to select "Air Fry" mode.
8. Press "Time Button" and again turn the dial to set the cooking time to 10 minutes.
9. Now push "Temp Button" and rotate the dial to set the temperature at 280 degrees F.
10. Press "Start/Pause" button to start.
11. When the unit beeps to show that it is preheated, open the lid.
12. Arrange the banana slices into the air fry basket and sprinkle with cinnamon sugar.
13. Insert the basket in the oven.
14. When cooking time is complete, open the lid and transfer the banana slices onto plates to cool slightly
15. Sprinkle with chopped walnuts and serve.
16. Serving Suggestions: Serve with a scoop of strawberry ice cream.
17. Variation Tip: Pecans will be an excellent substitute for walnuts.

Nutrition Info: Calories: 216 Fat: 8.8g Sat Fat: 5.3g Carbohydrates: 26g Fiber: 2.3g Sugar: 11.9g Protein: 3.4g

Gluten-free Cherry Crumble

Servings: 4
Cooking Time: 25 Minutes

Ingredients:
- 3 cups pitted cherries
- 2 teaspoons of lemon juice
- 1/3 cup butter
- 1 cup gluten-free all-purpose baking flour
- 1 teaspoon vanilla powder
- 10 tablespoons of white sugar

Directions:
1. Cube the butter and refrigerate for about 15 minutes. It should get firm.
2. Preheat your air fryer to 165 degrees C or 325 degrees F.
3. Bring together the pitted cherries, lemon juice, and 2 tablespoons of sugar in your bowl. Mix well.
4. Pour the cherry mix into a baking dish.
5. Now mix 6 tablespoons of sugar and flour in a bowl.
6. Use your fingers to cut in the butter. Particles should be pea-size.
7. Keep them over the cherries. Press down lightly.
8. Stir in the vanilla powder and 2 tablespoons of sugar in your bowl.
9. Dust the sugar topping over flour and cherries.
10. Transfer to your air fryer and bake.
11. Leave it inside for 10 minutes once the baking is done.
12. Set aside for 5 minutes to cool.

Nutrition Info: Calories 576, Carbohydrates 76g, Cholesterol 41mg, Total Fat 28g, Protein 5g, Sugar 49g, Fiber 6g, Sodium 109mg

Glazed Figs

Servings: 4
Cooking Time: 10 Minutes

Ingredients:
- 4 fresh figs
- 4 teaspoons honey
- 2/3 cup Mascarpone cheese, softened
- Pinch of ground cinnamon

Directions:
1. Cut each fig into the quarter, leaving just a little at the base to hold the fruit together.
2. Arrange the figs onto a parchment paper-lined sheet pan and drizzle with honey.
3. Place about 2 teaspoons of Mascarpone cheese in the center of each fig and sprinkle with cinnamon.
4. Press "Power Button" of Ninja Foodi Digital Air Fry Oven and turn the dial to select the "Air Broil" mode.
5. Press "Time Button" and again turn the dial to set the cooking time to 10 minutes.
6. Press "Start/Pause" button to start.
7. When the unit beeps to show that it is preheated, open the lid and insert the sheet pan in oven.
8. When cooking time is complete, open the lid and transfer the figs onto a platter.
9. Serve warm.
10. Serving Suggestions: Topping of chopped nuts will add a nice nutty texture.
11. Variation Tip: Select figs that are clean and dry, with smooth, unbroken skin.

Nutrition Info: Calories: 141 Fat: 5.5g Sat Fat: 3.5g Carbohydrates: 19.2g Fiber: 1.9g Sugar: 15g Protein: 5.3g